TREATING SPORTS INJURIES THE NATURAL WAY

TREATING
SPORTS
INJURIES
THE
NATURAL WAY

A homoeopathic self-treatment handbook

LYLE W. MORGAN II
Ph.D., H.M.D.

THORSONS PUBLISHING GROUP

This UK edition published 1990

First published 1988 by Healing Arts Press, Vermont, USA

British Library Cataloguing in Publication Data

Morgan, Lyle W.
Treating sports injuries the natural way
1. Sports. games. Sports & games injuries. Homeopathy.
remedies
I. Title
617'.1027

ISBN 0-7225-1604-5

*Published by Thorsons Publishers Limited,
Wellingborough, Northants NN8 2RQ, England*

Printed in Great Britain by Mackays of Chatham, Kent

1 3 5 7 9 10 8 6 4 2

To Harvey Neal Sievers, M.D., F.A.A.F.P., for his invaluable reading
of, and advice on the manuscript and for his unflagging desire to
be of service through friendship; for my father,
Lyle W. Morgan, who taught me that nothing is
impossible; and for Kevin Sean Anglen—best
friend, challenge, and inspiration.
With deep appreciation and affection.

A friend should be one in whose understanding and virtue we can
equally confide, and whose opinion we can value at once for its
justness and its sincerity.

—Robert Hall

ABOUT THE AUTHOR

Dr. Lyle W. Morgan II has been practising homeopathic medicine for more than 15 years. Holding a Ph.D. from the University of Nebraska, the Doctor of Medicine in Homoeopathy from the Université Internationale, Brux., and the distinction of Doctor of Nutritional Medicine from the John F. Kennedy College of Nutrimedical Arts & Sciences, he is currently serving as the Vice-President for Regional Operations of the American Nutritional Medical Association. Dr. Morgan holds membership in the American College of Natural Sports Medicine, and was recognized as a Fellow of the American Nutritional Medical Association in 1986. A healthcare educator and practitioner, he is also a professor and academic program director at Pittsburg State University, Pittsburg, Kansas.

CONTENTS

A READERS' ADVISORY

It is not the purpose or intent of this book to replace the professional services of a physician or sports medicine specialist. The reader should not hesitate to consult a physician, sports specialist, or other licensed health care practitioner for any illness or athletic injury that requires professional evaluation and treatment.

Homeotherapeutics have been used by physicians, licensed health care providers, and lay people for nearly two hundred years. Scientific research is now proving homeotherapeutics to have remarkable and valuable healing properties. Most homeopathic remedies are available as non-prescription, over-the-counter drugs with the exception of some tinctures, potencies, and special combinations that can be used only by licensed physicians.

The remedy indications and tables in this book have been taken from authoritative sources: the homeopathic *Materia Medica,* and the writings of physicians, clinicians, researchers, in scientific laboratory reports, medical documents, journals, and other related sources. No attempt should be made on the part of the reader to use any of this information as a form of treatment for illnesses or accidents that require the care of a licensed health care provider.

FOREWORD

We need this book.

While sports medicine has grown, with physicians trained in orthopedics now subspecializing in this area, practitioners have failed to take advantage of a wide variety of homeopathic remedies that are simple and effective when properly used. There has been an all-too-willing acceptance of "information" provided by drug companies concerning a small number of medications for sports-related physical problems – usually those on which a particular company holds patents. Rather, I'd like to see an exploration of the long-known and valuable healing properties of the various homeopathic remedies that Dr. Lyle Morgan now makes available. With these significant alternatives for healing sports-related injuries, Dr. Morgan fills a void in the literature and provides a much needed service to sports medicine for athletes, coaches, and trainers.

H. Neal Sievers, M.D., F.A.A.F.P.

PREFACE

People of every age the world over are participating in greater and greater numbers in an amazing array of athletic activities. They jog, walk, bicycle, hike, sail, water-ski, and lift weights. They play handball and squash, practice yoga, go camping. As their numbers increase, the number of athletic-related injuries continues to grow. Television and newspapers throughout the world lavish concern and interest on injured players, whether they be members of major athletic teams or students in school. Why then, I wonder, isn't equal attention given a soccer player at the Sportheim in Meyerhoffen, Austria, when he marches back into the field on the day following a sprained ankle, pulled hamstring, or bruised shin? Perhaps this apparent lack of interest comes as a result of people's familiarity with the rapid, near-magic cures that accrue in homeopathic medicine.

Since its discovery nearly two hundred years ago, by Samuel C. H. Hahnemann, a German physician and chemist, homeopathy has enjoyed widespread popularity and success both among the lay public and within a large and ever-growing number of the medical profession in England, France, and West Germany. In the Soviet Union, nearly one out of every three medical doctors is trained in homeopathy. This form of treatment has also found wide acceptance in India, which has more homeopathic medical colleges and hospitals than any other nation.

Up until the development of the so-called miracle drugs of sulfa and penicillin, homeopathy had enjoyed widespread acceptance in the United States, as well. Although the treatment has never ceased to be used entirely, it has, in recent times, begun to reassert itself more prominently as a viable and effective method of health care. Today, many young physicians are taking postgraduate studies in the homeotherapeutic method, and younger physicians are adding homeopathic remedies to their arsenals against illness, disease, and injury. As A. Dwight Smith, M.D., writes in *Homeopathy, A Rational and Scientific Method of Treatment,* "When a regular physician investigates homeopathy, he almost invariably adopts it." Homeopathy is accessible to the non-physician as well because, "With a minimum amount of homeopathic instruction, most trainers, coaches, and athletes themselves, can successfully treat and cure many of the most common athletic injuries. Their willingness to do so will have two results: quicker and more comfortable healing for the athlete; and thousands of dollars saved for the athletic club."[1]

Should the sporting public, trainers, and coaches then consider homeopathy as an effective treatment for minor athletic injuries? I'd answer that with an unqualified yes. Homeopathic medicines are nontoxic, and unlike most standard drugs and medications, do not have uncomfortable and/or dangerous side effects. Homeopathic remedies do not interact with other drugs the athlete may be taking, create no allergic reactions, and are always nonaddictive. They "usually cut healing time by 50–85 percent,"[2] and, because of their safety, the majority of homeopathic medicines are classified as nonprescription, over-the-counter drugs.

As demonstrated here and in the pages to follow, homeopathy offers a history strong in rapid healing incidence. There also can be little doubt that the homeopathic method is an excellent and inexpensive health care alternative. From the single dose of *Cuprum metallicum,* which relaxes severe muscular contractions in minutes, to *Symphytum,* given following a fracture, which, "usually cuts healing time by 50–75 percent,"[3] there can be no better way to manage sports, and other athlete-related illness.

Lyle W. Morgan II, H.M.D., Ph.D.

---

1. "Homeopathy and Sports Medicine," *American Homeopathy: Professional Edition,* Vol. 1, No. 6, June 1984, p. 50.

2. Ibid.

3. "Homeopathy and Sports Medicine," *American Homeopathy: Professional Edition,* Vol. 1, No. 6, June 1984, p. 5.

PART ONE

HOMEOPATHIC TREATMENT OF SPORTS INJURIES

CHAPTER ONE

THE ADVANTAGES OF HOMEOPATHIC TREATMENT

What does the sports-conscious homeopathic practitioner do for a middle-aged athlete with the vague complaint that her "knee hurts all the time"? This enthusiast enjoyed jogging and rapid walking for health and recreation, and had developed, four years earlier, a painful and essentially undiagnosed knee joint disorder. She went to a family physician who diagnosed "peri-articular arthritis" and recommended injections of the powerful adrenal corticosteroid, cortisone, to relieve the inflammation. The initial treatment worked, but the pain returned after only a few weeks. Yet another physician diagnosed "chondritis," an inflammation of the meniscus cartilage, and "tendinitis." Opposing cortisone as a "method of final treatment only," this doctor prescribed Motrin, a non-steroidal anti-inflammatory (NSAID) frequently prescribed for athletic injuries of the joints and inflammations of connective tissues. The Motrin "cut into [her] stomach like a knife" and she stopped taking it. Chiropractic manipulations had succeeded in reducing the overall discomfort, but the knee remained unstable, the pains radiating along the outside of the knee, requiring massage and constant supporting pressure.

In homeopathy there are no such things as "peri-articular arthritis," or "chondritis," or "tendinitis."

"The word 'homeopathy' is derived from the two Greek words, *homois* meaning similar and *pathos* meaning suffering, and their combination represents a very concise description of the homeopathic method of remedy selection. A remedy selected homeopathically is chosen because of its ability to produce in a healthy person a range of symptoms similar to that observed in the patient. In other words, the appropriate remedy, in effect, should be able to produce in a healthy person a similar type of suffering to that experienced by the patient."[4]

Returning to the middle-aged female athlete – for almost four years nothing in the arsenal of standard medical treatment had worked; the alternative therapy of chiropractic had helped, but not cured the condition. "Is there anything you can do?" she asked.

In the initial evaluative interview, which lasted over an hour, every symptom was presented in the woman's own words: "It aches like a toothache, constantly. . . . It's always better when I rub it. . . . I can only walk downstairs sideways, and put both feet on each step, or I'm afraid I'll fall over." She was asked a great many questions: "Is the pain constant, or does it come and go?" (The pain was always worse on first movement and became less noticeable with continued movement. If she rose from the bed, the knee hurt; if she got up from a chair, the knee hurt. But continued movement was less distressing.) "Is the pain worse or better in cold weather?" (Here the knee always ached and throbbed in cold weather and was even worse in cold dampness.)

As he views patients, the homeopathic practitioner must consider a myriad of details, among them, a review of the more than 2,000 remedies in the *Materia Medica,* where hundreds of thousands of symptomatic complaints are discussed. He has to focus on *mentalities* – the psychological and emotional state of the patient. He needs to look at *acute symptoms* – the exact nature of the overall symptoms, major and minor, that the patient experiences, and *modalities* – those symptoms brought about by outside factors, which still play an important part in the disease. Special attention has to be given to those factors influencing the condition itself. Is it made better as a result of movement, or worse because of it? Does the problem become worse as a result of rest, or better when it is exercised? Does cold or warmth play a role in the nature of the complaint?

Then the practitioner must find out when the complaint appeared, and for how long it has existed. An *acute condition* is one that has only begun recently, whereas *chronic condition* is one that has existed for a period of weeks, months, or even years. Another description is that of *constitutional condition*, a specific symptom complex found from generation to generation in some families that predisposes their members to severe diseases such as cancer or tuberculosis.

After a close study of all the aspects of the patient and of the disease process, the homeopathic practitioner begins the task of eliminating those symptoms that the patient—and the symptom pictures of the remedies—do not produce. He needs to find one, perhaps two or three remedies, that most closely match the nature of the patient's Keynote symptoms. With these in place, the appropriate potency of the chosen remedy can be prescribed. Generally, in acute illnesses or injuries, lower potencies are selected.[5] In long-standing conditions, the chronic conditions, high potencies are most frequently employed.

Based on homeopathic analysis, the athlete's condition was a chronic symptom, joint pain in the knee; her modalities, better from movement and supporting pressure, better from massage, better from warmth, and worse from cold and damp; and her mentality, frequently tired and listless—a symptom she had not volunteered during the initial interview, but which had been observed in her continual sighing, slumping posture, and which was questioned. The symptoms taken together dictated one specific remedy: *Rhus toxicodendron*, commonly called *Rhus tox.*, a homeopathic polycrest prepared from the poison ivy plant.

The homeopathic method was methodically determined in clinical studies through the use of "provers," healthy people who lent themselves to experiments in which they were given specific plant, animal, and mineral substances that produced specific illnesses or symptoms, which were carefully recorded by homeopathic researchers. The underlying theory is best explained as: "If all the known drugs and many more could be 'proved' on healthy people, then the resulting drug pictures would supply specific and accurate indications for their use. One would simply have to match a patient's symptom picture with an appropriate drug picture."[6] And the theory works. Homeopathy alone among the many schools of health care—standard medicine, allopathy (meaning *allos*, "other," and *pathos*, "suffering"), osteopathy, chiropractic, and naturopathy—has remained virtually untouched by continuous change. It is indeed difficult and certainly nonsensical to tamper with a system of health care that works, and works consistently.

For the female athlete, due to the nature of her condition (no specific diagnosis was made or attempted), *Rhus tox.* was clearly indicated. However, because of the longevity of the condition (its chronic nature), a high-potency remedy was selected – the 200c. She was directed to take a single unit dose of *Rhus tox.* 200c once every other day for a total of two doses, then stop the remedy for a week, then repeat the treatment as before, and await results.

Three days following the initial therapy, the woman returned. A smile lined her face where earlier there had been a consistent downward slope about the mouth. "Do you notice anything different?" she asked. And, without giving an opportunity for response, she exclaimed, "I am walking down the stairs like a normal person, and the pain is gone."

In homeopathy there is a vital principle. When a remedy, well selected based on the Keynote symptoms, produces a beneficial result, all further treatment ceases. The athlete was directed to discontinue the two-week course of therapy and to repeat it only if symptoms recurred. This case was treated in midsummer 1984. Almost two years and six months later, the woman has experienced no further recurrence of the condition.

In the late summer of 1984, a man with an athletic injury came for homeopathic evaluation and treatment. A university professor, he was age 42, and an active summertime softball player. During the rest of the year, he was essentially sedentary. He complained of a severely painful and debilitating shoulder injury. He had visited his own physician, a general internist, some four weeks earlier, and was given the diagnosis of "tendinitis," and a nonsteroidal anti-inflammatory drug had been prescribed. But the drug, while eliminating the pain during treatment, failed to provide permanent relief. When the prescription was exhausted, the pain returned. The professor, Dr. Michael H., was in continual discomfort, and was forced to discontinue playing softball. The shoulder throbbed and ached. The pain became worse with all movement, better at rest and with the cessation of movement, but worse from pressure. He could not sleep on the injured side; he could not place any weight against it by leaning on the elbow of the affected shoulder; nor could he raise his arm above shoulder height without excruciating pain. His physician had told him that eventually the injury would resolve itself. That, however, would not be for many weeks. In the meantime, additional medication could be prescribed. Understandably, the professor desired a more immediate relief, and something that would allow him to complete the softball season.

Observing closely the two cases presented here, the two complaints are clinically similar. Both complained of joint pain, one of the knee, the other of the shoulder. To standard medical practice, both conditions were almost entirely similar and both individuals had been prescribed the same anti-inflammatory, Motrin. But, homeopathically, both athletes had totally different Keynote symptoms. In the first case, beginning movement aggravated the pain, but continued movement lessened it. In the second case, the symptoms were reversed. In the first case, pressure and massage improved the pain; in the second, pressure increased it. To the homeopathically trained practitioner, the athletes had totally different disorders.

The softball-playing professor's remedy was *Bryonia,* the homeopathic preparation of the wild hops plant. And, since the nature of his condition had continued for only several weeks, it was considered acute rather than chronic, and a lower, mid-range potency of *Bryonia* was suggested, to be taken in five 1-grain tablet doses every 4 hours until the majority of painful symptoms subsided, at which point the healing process had begun and treatment would be discontinued.

To the nonhomeopathically trained individual, the rapidity at which homeopathic remedies frequently work can indeed be dazzling.

In the first case presented, a disorder which had lasted nearly four years was resolved without further treatment within a week. In the second case, and admittedly to the surprise of both patient and practitioner, the initial, in-house dosage of *Bryonia* produced such an immediate relief of pain that the patient was actually leaning heavily against the elbow of his injured shoulder, ten to fifteen minutes following medication. At that point pain was still present, but bearable. The discomfort ended, and total mobility of the shoulder returned, within several days of treatment. Such immediate healings under homeopathic care are not uncommon in the management of sports injuries.

Homeopathy as a system of health care treatment offers athletes, trainers, coaches, and all other interested individuals a number of positive advantages over any other known form of treatment for the most common injuries and illnesses.

1. INDIVIDUALIZATION. Homeopathic treatment is directed entirely at the individual; his or her acute or chronic symptoms, mentalities, and modalities of the disease process. Treatment is not directed toward a specific diagnostic disease name, but at the individual who is a unique biological and psychological entity ("He may not have the disease suspected."[7])

2. DRUG PROVING. Homeopathic experimentation and proving has, from the inception of this health care system, relied entirely on human experiment. Unlike allopathic drugs, homeopathic remedies are not tested on animals to determine effectiveness and reliability before they are made available to people.

3. HOMEOPATHIC METHOD. Homeopathy uses the *totality* of Keynote symptoms in the treatment of injuries and illness. At the same time, homeopathy directs its treatment at *cure,* not merely the palliation (lessening) of the disease process. Aspirin masks a headache and codeine masks a cough, but neither drug cures the underlying cause. Homeopathy directs a biological treatment that assists the body to remove the *cause* of the disease process and therefore provide a cure.

4. THE TEST OF TIME. Homeopathy is the only system of health care that by the uniqueness of its approach to health, has withstood the test of time. For nearly 200 years, thousands of physicians and millions of patients have clearly demonstrated homeopathy's success. "Medical fads, fakes, and delusions always run a course and are forgotten — not so with homeopathy. It is ethically practiced today by physicians who have studied it and many more who have taken postgraduate courses."[8]

5. WITHOUT SIDE EFFECTS. Unlike allopathic drugs, the majority of which, because of their possible, and potentially serious, side effects, are available only on a physician's prescription, homeopathic remedies have no side effects, produce no adverse drug interactions, are nonallergenic, and create no harmful or annoying after effects.

6. LOW COST AND EASE OF APPLICATION. Homeopathic remedies are available at very reasonable cost. This is because they are not patented. Homeopathic pharmaceutical manufacturers are not, therefore, required by economics to recover hundreds of millions of dollars in research costs, nor desirous of high profit margins like the allopathic drug industry. Any physician, any athlete, coach, or trainer who is will-

ing to study the basic tenets of homeotherapeutics can, with confidence, employ homeopathic remedies without potential danger, and with the reasonable assurance of success.

7. NO EXPIRATION DATE. Homeopathic remedies, unlike allopathic pharmaceuticals—when stored and treated properly—do not lose their potency or change their chemical composition.

---

4. Keith A. Scott, M.B., & Linda A. McCourt, M.A., *Homeopathy: The Potent Force of the Minimum Dose* (Wellingborough, Northamptonshire, England: Thorsons Publishers, Ltd., 1982), p. 11.

5. Potencies and their selection will be presented at a later point in this book.

6. Scott & McCourt, *op. cit.*, p. 21.

7. Garth W. Boericke, M.D., "Some Advantages of Homeopathy," *American Homeopathy*, Vol. 1, No. 2, September 1984, p. 17.

8. Ibid.

CHAPTER TWO

HOW HOMEOPATHIC REMEDIES ARE MANUFACTURED

There exists a considerable difference between homeopathic remedies and the more common allopathic pharmaceuticals. Homeopathic remedies are actually system stimulators—products that, by their nature, act upon the body's own natural defense mechanism against the disease process to bring about healing. They are to be dispensed for brief periods. Allopathic pharmaceuticals act against the disease process more directly than do homeopathic remedies. They are prescribed for periods of from one to several weeks, and in relatively massive doses, as for example, Keflex (an antibiotic), 250 mg; Chlorpropamide (a drug to treat diabetes), 250 mg; Ketoprofen (an anti-inflammatory), 75 mg.

The human body's immune system is still not well understood by medical science. In formulating or prescribing remedies for various illnesses, conventional medicine has concentrated on specific organisms (bacteria, viruses) and hormonal imbalances that create diseases or syndromes. While homeopathy has always recognized these factors, it has also spoken of the mind-spirit-body connection, and the underlying vital life force. Because of its almost mystical connotation, the term "vital life force" has created some confusion about the homeopathic view of health. However, put simply, the vital life force provides the resiliency, flexibility, and ability to adapt to circumstances that we experience in our daily lives when under stress—such as changes in climate or diet, illness, grief, or even travel. This vital life force is an integral part of the mind-spirit-body connection, and modern science is beginning to explain such aspects of homeopathy in its own terms.

"Until recently, [homeopathic] physicians have been unable to explain the mechanism involved in the healing effect of their particular practice. Today's physicist can explain the mechanism of action of both acupuncture and homeopathy. Medicines in homeopathy are often diluted beyond the existence of a single atom of the original substance. The unique energy field of a substance, the magnetic blueprint, maintains its identity in the absence of that substance in a material sense. Indeed, the less of a material substance present, the greater the intensity of the magnetic field and the greater or more profound is the effect upon the body."[9]

Homeopathy does not rely on dosages of substances in the tens and hundreds of milligrams.

The process involved in the manufacture of homeopathic remedies and their various potencies is far too complex to consider here in any depth. It should suffice to say that plant, mineral, and animal substances pass through a process which produces a *dilution* (in the case of substances soluble in alcohol and water) or a *trituration* (in the case of certain minerals which are nonsoluble). From the base substance, through a complex manufacturing process, the various *potencies* of homeopathic remedies are made.

There exist two systems of determining the potency of remedies, the *decimal* and the *centesimal* scales. Homeopathic potencies most commonly available in the United States are produced on the decimal scale. Here, one part of the base substance that will become a homeopathic remedy is added to nine parts of the diluting medium—for soluble substances, alcohol and water, for nonsoluble substances, lactose. This creates the *first*, or 1x potency. Successive potencies are made by adding one part of the first potency to nine parts of diluting medium and so on. At each stage in the dilution process, the potencies are shaken vigorously to create the "magnetic blueprint" that differentiates homeopathic remedies from allopathic pharmaceuticals. The centesimal scale, more common in Europe and other parts of the world, is produced in the same fashion but adds one part of base substance to 99 parts of diluting medium. This creates the 1c potency.

Unfortunately, an absolute standard to designate homeopathic potencies does not appear to exist. Decimal potencies are most frequently designated as 1x, 2x, 3x, etc., but in some cases as 1D, 2D, 3D. They are the same potency whatever the notation system. The centesimal scale is most commonly written as 1, 2, 3, etc., but sometimes appears as 1c, 2c, and 3c or 1cH, 2cH, 3cH, indicating "Centesimal Hahnemann" in honor of Samuel Hahnemann, the founder of homeopathy. Below is a table that compares the actual dilution ratio of the decimal and centesimal scales.

DILUTION RATIO	DECIMAL SCALE (x)	CENTESIMAL SCALE (c)
1/10 or 10^{-1}	1x	—
1/100 or 10^{-2}	2x	1c
1/1000 or 10^{-3}	3x	—
1/10000 or 10^{-4}	4x	2c
10^{-6}	6x	3c
10^{-12}	12x	6c
10^{-24}	24x	12c
10^{-30}	30x	15c
10^{-60}	60x	30c
10^{-2000}	—	M (1000c)
10^{-20000}	—	10M (10000c)
$10^{-200000}$	—	CM (100000c)

In the standard practice of homeopathy, only licensed health care professionals employ potencies above 200x or 200c. Clinical practice and recent research studies conducted at major medical schools and research institutions are beginning to explain the nature of the effectiveness of homeopathic micro-dilutions. Homeopathic practitioners have found, through continued application of homeopathic potencies, that the *higher* the potency (that is, the more the basic substance is diluted and potentized), the more dynamically reactive it is in the body. This may seem contrary to our understanding of dilution when dealing with medicines, but it is, in fact, how homeopathy works. Homeopaths have also found that the centesimal scale of dilution produces remedies that are more vitally reactive in the body than those produced on the decimal scale. For example the 6c potency is more reactive than the 6x, the 30c more potent than the 30x, etc. In general, the most commonly used decimal potencies are the 3x, 6x, and 30x and, on the centesimal scale, the 3c, 6c, and 15c potencies. The lower numbers represent the *lower* potencies (3x/c, 6x/c) the two-digit numbers the *mid-range* potencies (12x/c, 30x/c), and the numbers of three digits the *high* potencies (200x/c) The *highest* homeopathic potencies employ the Roman numeral designation of M (1000); a number plus a numeral, 10M (10,000); or a combination of Roman numerals, CM (100,000).

ADVISORY WARNING: Homeopathic potencies above the 200c (usually written as 200) should be used only by the health care professional who is highly trained in homeotherapeutics. The use of the highest potencies is, as the famous American homeopathic physician once said, like balancing on a razor's keen edge. Homeopathic high potencies are so dynamically potent that they have the power to stimulate the immuno-defense system so quickly and with such violence as to require only the skilled physician to safely administer them. [10]

---

9. *Journal of Ultramolecular Medicine* (Provo, UT: Brigham Young University, 1983), Vol. 1, No. 1, p. 42.

10. Elizabeth Wright-Hubbard, M.D.. *A Brief Study Course in Homeopathy* (St. Louis: Formur, Inc., 1977).

CHAPTER THREE

HOMEOPATHIC COMBINATION REMEDIES

"Homeopathy . . . does not promote one approach to homeopathy over another.

Qualified, competent people differ in their professional beliefs as to which approach to the homeopathic system is most appropriate or works the best. That minds differ in no way affects the credibility of homeopathy. Rather, such interplay, we believe, prompts practitioners to apply their art more consciously and more effectively, constantly stimulated by the ideas and experiences of their peers."[11]

Traditionally, homeopathy attempts to direct a *single,* most appropriate remedy to target the disease process as experienced in an illness or injury. Classical homeopathy firmly believes that, in the 2,000 or more remedies available, and keynoted in an expanse of major and minor symptom pictures, there are single remedies that specifically "target" particular diseases or injuries. However, homeopathic practitioners vary considerably in their application of the science and art of homeotherapeutics. Some practitioners are "low potency" prescribers, employing remedies in potencies below 15c or 30x. Other homeopaths are "high potency" prescribers, utilizing only the highest homeopathic potencies (200, M, 10M, 50M, and CM). Still others, both physicians and homeopathic practitioners, prefer to use varying potencies from tinctures (an alcohol and water extract of a soluble substance at one-tenth its crude strength, symbolized by 0) through to the highest designations. They use as their guide the process of the disease itself, and the unique, biological and psychological makeup of the patient.

There are many applications of homeopathy, yet overall, the system of homeotherapeutics – the nature of the remedies and the remedies themselves – remains unchanged. Though not an altogether new practice, homeopathic practitioners have recently been developing and dispensing more combination remedies. Actually, many homeopathic pharmaceutical manufacturers have for decades produced special "house" combinations, using two, three, and sometimes as many as four or five compatible remedies. These combinations, proven over time through clinical practice and application, have permitted the homeopathic prescriber to cover a broader range of symptoms, in a more rapid manner, than is generally possible in the selection of a single remedy.

"Combination remedies are mixtures of two or more homeopathic ingredients of the same or different attenuations. These combinations are designed by physicians or pharmacists with extensive knowledge of the *Materia Medica*. Ingredients are selected for combination based on the purpose of the remedy and therefore may be few or many depending upon the complexity desired. Ingredients which are related in their symptom 'pictures' for a particular condition are assembled to broaden the total 'picture' for the combination remedy. Combined ingredients which mutually support or reinforce each other's effects provide the prescriber with a simple means of treating common acute conditions. By combining several ingredients' 'pictures' into a single broader remedy it is not necessary for the prescriber to have an extensive knowledge of the *Materia Medica* or to select the exactly matching single remedy. While combination remedies are not often used in treatment of chronic or constitutional cases, they are frequently used to treat the acute symptoms accompanying the condition, or to clarify the constitutional condition by removing acute symptoms. This last is done because the acute symptoms may cloud the constitutional 'picture' and make it difficult to distinguish.

It is true that treatment with single remedies that are the exact similia for the patient is always the best possible treatment. Not every prescriber, however, will have the expertise or time to discern this exact remedy in every case, nor is it always necessary. The practitioner today is called upon to treat so many patients for such a broad range of conditions, the majority of which are acute and common, that this is simply not practical. The value of combination homeopathic remedies is best utilized for these most common conditions."[12]

This book contains dozens of homeopathic single remedies, together with their most common Keynote symptom pictures, to cover the many common and uncommon physical complaints athletes may experience. The use of special combination remedies, however, is encouraged, especially for the athlete, trainer, sports coach, or physician who is learning about the homeopathic method. The combinations currently available from the majority of homeopathic pharmaceutical houses and pharmacies are exceptionally effective and reliable.

ADVISORY WARNING: No attempt should be made by the nonphysician or pharmacist to combine single homeopathic remedies. Some remedies are incompatible in combination and antidote one another. Combination remedies should be used only as delivered by a reliable homeopathic pharmacist, or chemist.

---

11. "Is There Just One Approach to Homeopathy?", *American Homeopathy,* Vol. 1, No. 2, September, 1984, p. 12.

12. *Homeopathic Therapy Physicians' Reference* (Biological Homeopathic Industries, Albuquerque, NM, MENACO Publishing Company, Inc., 1986), pp. 2-3.

CHAPTER FOUR

THE PRACTICE OF HOMEOPATHY

The athlete, trainer, coach, or physician who is studying and using homeotherapeutics as a viable treatment method for common injuries and illnesses needs to be apprised of what not to do when using homeopathic remedies.

The following statements are guidelines for the correct application of homeopathic remedies:

1. Select the one single remedy that *most* specifically covers the majority ("totality") of symptoms the patient is currently experiencing, using the Keynote symptoms presented in this book, or in a homeopathic *Materia Medica* with repertory. Or use a combination remedy recommended for the problem being experienced.

2. Do not continue to take, or administer, homeopathic remedies indefinitely. The vital principle in homeopathy is to stop taking or giving a remedy whenever there is no sign of improvement; or there is a definite improvement in the condition being treated. The continued use of homeopathic remedies under either condition is both wasteful and ill-advised. Whenever a remedy best indicated fails to work (rare), it is the incorrect remedy for the condition. Here the practitioner reexamines the Keynote symptoms to find the correct remedy. Whenever a definite

improvement in symptoms occurs, the single remedy or combination is stopped. Healing has already been established, signalling no further need for medication.

3. Avoid using potencies above the 200 designation and only that potency as directed in this book for specially indicated circumstances. The use of high and highest potency remedies is dangerous and ill-advised for anyone other than an experienced physician or licensed health care practitioner. The nonphysician/practitioner should employ only the midrange and lower potencies. Combination remedies never exceed the 30th potency of any one of the remedies.

4. Nonphysicians/practitioners must limit their use of homeopathic remedies to *acute* conditions only and make no attempt to treat either chronic or constitutional conditions.

5. Do not handle the remedies needlessly. Remedies should be transferred directly from their container into the cap of that container (in the case of tablets and pills or pellets) or as drops directly into the mouth. Handling of homeopathic remedies can cause contamination and loss of potency.

6. The majority of homeopathic remedies are taken by mouth. Because of their unique chemical nature, tablets or drops are placed directly *under the tongue* (sublingually) where they are rapidly absorbed into the bloodstream through the capillaries that line the mucous membranes of the mouth and act as sponges for medications. *Unless specifically directed, remedies are never swallowed.*

7. When taking homeopathic remedies, care must be observed to *avoid* drinking coffee, tea, or any beverage containing caffeine. In some persons, these beverages appear to nullify the effectiveness of the remedy.

8. Maintain a "clean" mouth while taking remedies. *Do not use* mouthwash or toothpaste for at least 30–60 minutes before, or after, taking a homeopathic remedy. The mint flavoring contained in most mouthwashes and toothpastes will nullify some remedies. It is best not to eat at least 15–30 minutes before, or after, taking any remedy.

9. Keep all remedies away from direct sunlight, and avoid exposing remedies to strong-smelling perfumes and household cleaning products.

Keep containers tightly capped, and do not open more than one container of a remedy in the presence of another remedy (to avoid cross-contamination).

These simple recommendations for the proper use of homeopathic remedies will assist in ensuring success in treatment.

Because of the low cost of homeopathic remedies, should a remedy be suspected of contamination, it is best to discard it and purchase a fresh supply.

PART TWO

GENERAL MEDICAL PROBLEMS IN SPORTS

CHAPTER FIVE

EYE PROBLEMS

Topics Covered

Mechanical Injuries: Black Eye
Mechanical Injuries: Foreign Objects in the Eye
Subconjunctival Hemorrhage
Conjunctivitis
Sty
Inflammation of the Eyelid: Blepharitis
Wounds of the Eye
Concurrent Homeopathic Remedies in Eye Inflammations

Mechanical Injuries: Black Eye

The so-called black eye, a bruise, really, is not an injury to the eye itself but to the eye's surrounding tissues. Usually the result of a blow from a hard object or fist, the black eye is a rupture of the small blood vessels in the delicate tissues of the eyelid, or the tissue surrounding the eye.

HOMEOPATHIC TREATMENT
Arnica Montana
Ledum Palustre (Ledum Pal.)
Symphytum Officinale (Symphytum Off.)

23

Arnica is the preeminent remedy in homeopathy for the repair of damaged blood vessels. Known as a short-acting but rapidly effective remedy, Arnica brings about a rapid resolution of pain and the bruised feeling and swelling from a black eye.

Potency and Dosage: 6x–30x or 30c, three doses, one every 30 minutes, then three doses three times a day for one to three days.

Ledum Pal. is almost specific for any bruising injury where there is the traditional black and blue or purplish discoloration of the skin. Ledum pal. particularly relates to the discoloration itself (produced by the effusion of blood from the ruptured vessels into the surrounding tissues) and when the modality "better from cold application" is present. Therefore, if the black eye feels better from placing a cold cloth over it, Ledum pal. would be the remedy of choice. Ledum pal. brings about a rapid reabsorption of the blood, reduction of swelling, and the return of normal skin coloration.

ADVISORY WARNING: Never apply a source of cold directly to the eye. Ice cubes or cold packs should be wrapped in a cloth before being placed against the eye.

Potency and Dosage: 6x–30x or 30c, three doses, one every 30 minutes, then three doses three times a day for one to three days.

Symphytum is best used if there has been direct injury to the eyeball itself, and when pain is present. Symphytum is best alternated with Arnica in treating this injury.

Potency and Dosage: 6x–30x or 30c, three doses, one every 30 minutes. Stop Symphytum and proceed with Arnica in the same potency, one dose every 30 minutes for three doses, then three doses three times a day for one to three days.

ADVISORY WARNING: If the eye itself has been injured by a direct blow from a hard object such as a fist, tennis or raquette ball, baseball or softball, the patient must be taken to a physician or hospital emergency room for proper medical evaluation. This is especially true if the victim complains of severe pain in the eye, double vision, and/or if there is obvious bleeding inside the anterior chamber of the eyeball.

Mechanical Injuries: Foreign Objects in the Eye

Jogging and outdoor sporting play often cause particles of dust, dirt, or grit to enter the eye. It is not uncommon for base runners to experience this, or for a jogger to have a small insect fly into the eye. The foreign object irritates the eye and causes burning, itching, and, perhaps, a localized redness. These symptoms are accompanied by intense watering, the eye's natural defense as it attempts to cleanse itself.

Taking this cue from nature, when a foreign object enters the eye, try to flush it free, by rinsing with cool water. You can use any brand of eyedrops, as well. Most people find the process uncomfortable, because the anticipation of anything entering the eye produces a lid-shutting reflex. Do continue to work the lid open. Often, flushing alone will remove the object. However, if adequate flushing fails, or the object becomes trapped underneath the lid, use a clean, damp piece of cloth, tissue, or cotton swab and gently touch it against the object. It should adhere and can then be easily removed. If the object is trapped under the lid itself, roll the lid back against the support of a cotton-tipped swab and remove the object. The lid will fold back easily against support.

HOMEOPATHIC TREATMENT

Irritation of the eye, that annoying itch, can continue for some time following the object's removal. If this is true, flush the eye with a solution of pure water to which 2–3 drops of *Calendula Succus* or *Tincture, Hypericum* or *Euphrasia Tincture* has been added. Such local treatment using homeopathic liquid remedies will quickly cure the irritation.

> ADVISORY WARNING: Never attempt to remove any object that has become embedded in the surface of the eye. Embedded glass, gravel, rush, cigarette ash, slivers, comprise a medical emergency that requires the physician's expertise.

If medical help is not immediately available, do the following first aid:

1. If at all possible, cover the injured eye with a paper cup and bandage the cup in place. If this is not available, cover the eye with a bandage, being careful not to exert any pressure against the eye.
2. Since eyes move in tandem, it is best to cover *both* eyes.
3. If available, give one dose of Arnica in 30x, 30c, or 200c potency. Arnica acts as a sedative against pain and will help promote healing.

4. Take the victim as quickly as possible to the nearest physician or hospital emergency room where the embedded object will be removed and the injury properly treated.

Subconjunctival Hemorrhage

Though greatly alarming for most people, the subconjunctival hemorrhage is not dangerous. It can be caused by hard coughing or sneezing and, occasionally, by lifting weights. The condition can also come without any apparent precipitating cause.

Subconjunctival hemorrhaging is the spontaneous rupture of tiny blood vessels in the sclera or "white" of the eye. The sclera will be greatly inflamed or nearly completely red. The condition is self-limiting, lasting from 5 to 14 days. The eye heals itself without medical treatment. It is not uncommon for there to be a rebleed on the fifth day.

Homeopathic treatment, however, almost always produces a permanent resolution within 12 to 24 hours in subconjunctival hemorrhage.

HOMEOPATHIC TREATMENT
Arnica Montana
Hamamelis
Ledum Palustre (Ledum Pal.)

Arnica is often the first remedy considered in treating a subconjunctival hemorrhage because of its ability to rapidly reabsorb blood from leaking vessels and to quickly repair them.

Potency and Dosage: 6x–30x or 30c, one dose every 3 to 4 hours until the condition noticeably improves. The 200c potency should act especially rapidly, usually in 12 to 24 hours.

Hamamelis, a homeopathic remedy made from the shrub witch hazel, known for its astringent properties, is frequently the most effective treatment of subconjunctival hemorrhage. Hamamelis has the power to rapidly reabsorb blood and seal off further leaking. It is most often called upon as a secondary remedy to Arnica, but might well be considered first. Hamamelis usually brings about complete recovery within 24 hours.

Potency and Dosage: 6x–30x or 30c, one dose every 3 to 4 hours until the condition noticeably improves. The 200c potency should act especially rapidly, usually in 12 to 24 hours.

Ledum Pal. is a third homeopathic remedy to consider in subconjunctival hemorrhage, when the condition has the appearance of an extravasation of blood beneath the sclera (white), sometimes accompanied by a mild aching.

Potency and Dosage: 6x–30x or 30c, one dose every 3 to 4 hours as needed until improvement sets in. The 200c potency should act especially rapidly, usually in 12 to 24 hours.

> ADVISORY WARNING: A subconjunctival hemorrhage can be differentiated from another, more serious injury by the fact that there is no history of traumatic injury to the eye. If the eye itself has been injured by a direct blow from a hard object, the patient must always be taken to a physician or hospital emergency room for proper medical evaluation and treatment.

Conjunctivitis

This greatly annoying eye condition is not an uncommon occurrence in athletes. It is most often caused by either a bacterial or a viral infection, or by allergy. Sometimes, however, the cause is mechanical – such as a foreign object, or a chemical irritant in the eye.

The causal factor of conjunctivitis is easy to determine, although in homeopathy the totality of Keynote symptoms is more important in determining effective treatment than is the cause of the condition.

Bacterial conjunctivitis is the most common form of the condition. It produces a purulent discharge from the eye often accompanied by a mild swelling of the lid. Usually a self-limiting condition, it will resolve in 10 to 14 days. Viral conjunctivitis produces a clear discharge from the eye (the opposite of bacterial infection). There may be mild lid swelling, but no itching. In irritation from allergy, there may be clear or stringy discharge from the eye, accompanied by moderate to severe swelling of the lid and intense itching.

Aside from the above causes, irritation of the conjunctiva may follow exposure to air pollutants, such as wind, air-borne dust particles, bright and reflected light such as fishermen may experience off the water if they fail to wear sunglasses.

Conjunctivitis of nearly any cause is almost always self-limiting even without medical intervention. Bacterial conjunctivitis will usually resolve itself in 10 to 14 days, or 2 to 3 with antibiotic treatment. The homeopathic treatment of the condition is most often effective in 2 to 3 days as well. Viral conjunctivitis will usually clear without treatment in 1 to 3 weeks. Antibiotics are ineffective in treating a viral inflammation, and it is in virus-caused irritation where homeopathic treatment most often shows its true power. Without treatment, allergic conjunctivitis will continue until the causative factor is removed or the underlying allergy properly treated.

HOMEOPATHIC TREATMENT
Aconite
Arnica Montana
Arsenicum Album (Arsenicum Alb.)
Belladonna
Euphrasia
Pulsatilla
Sulphur

Each of the remedies listed above is specific to acute conjunctivitis regardless of the cause. The selection of the most effective remedy must, however, be made according to the overall Keynote symptoms the athlete is showing.

Aconite is appropriate under the following symptoms:

1. Eyes are red and inflamed.
2. Eyes feel dry and hot; gritty as if sand were trapped under the lids.
3. Lids are swollen, hard, and red.
4. The athlete has a great aversion to light of all kinds, to glare and to reflection.
5. Eyes water profusely after exposure to cold dry wind.

Potency and Dosage: 6x–30x or 30c, one dose every 3 to 4 hours until a noticeable improvement of the condition is seen.

Arnica is especially useful in eye irritation of a mechanical cause, where there is redness, heat, and swelling accompanied by a bruised, sore feeling.

Arsenicum Alb. is appropriate under the following conditions:

1. Eyes burn with an acidlike watering and tearing.
2. Lids are red, and appear granulated or ulcerated, scabby and scaly.
3. Lids are swollen and there is puffiness around the eyes.
4. Watering and tearing is burning and hot.
5. Lids are extremely painful.
6. The athlete experiences an intense aversion to all light, natural or artificial.

Potency and Dosage: 6x–30x or 30c, one dose every 3 to 4 hours as needed until a noticeable improvement sets in.

Belladonna is a preeminent eye remedy, special for the intensity and violence of its Keynote symptoms:

1. Eyes feel swollen, often as if they were bulging outward.
2. The conjunctiva is red, dry, and burning.
3. Lids are greatly swollen.
4. The athlete experiences throbbing or shooting pains in the affected eye.
5. There is a definite aversion to light.

Potency and Dosage: 6x–30x or 30c, one dose every 3 to 4 hours as needed until there is noticeable lessening of the condition.

Euphrasia is prepared homeopathically from the herb eyebright and is considered one of the most valuable of all eye remedies. Euphrasia's special value is in eye irritations of allergic origin. The remedy may be used effectively either in its tableted form or in a liquid preparation. Externally,

Euphrasia may be applied locally by diluting 2 to 3 drops of the tincture in an eye cup of distilled water and the affected eye(s) flushed with the solution several times a day. This is greatly soothing, especially in the allergic condition.

1. The discharge from the eye(s) is acidic and thick.
2. Eyelids are swollen and burn.
3. The athlete has a frequent desire to blink and the eyes water constantly.
4. There is an intense aversion to light, especially to artificial indoor lighting.
5. Small blisters may form on the cornea.

Potency and Dosage: 3x, 6x or 3c potency is preferred in Euphrasia, with one dose given every 2 to 3 hours and repeated as often as needed until there is a noticeable improvement in the overall condition. Lower homeopathic potencies bear more frequent repetition and may be used for a longer period than the higher potencies.

Pulsatilla is appropriate under the following circumstances:

1. The eye(s) produces a thick, profuse, yellow, and nonacidic discharge.
2. The discharge is accompanied by itching and burning.
3. Watering and tearing are profuse.
4. The eye(s) feels worse from warmth.
5. Lids are inflamed and the eye is closed shut with a sticky mucus.

Potency and Dosage: 6x–30x or 30c, one dose every 3 to 4 hours as needed until a definite improvement in overall symptoms is noted.

Sulphur is an especially useful remedy in any chronic inflammation of the eyelids whenever there is its characteristic burning, especially of the lid margins. Sulphur follows well in acute eye disorders, when soreness continues even after Arnica or Aconite have been used. In chronic eye inflammations Sulphur follows Arsenicum Album well when the irritation continues, but no acute inflammation is present. There are the following symptoms:

1. Burning of the margins or the eyelids.
2. The athlete experiences a feeling of heat and burning in the eyes. (Compare Arsenicum Album and Belladonna.)
3. Eyes itch and burn constantly.

Potency and Dosage: 6x–30x or 30c, one dose every 3 to 4 hours as needed until a definite improvement in overall symptoms is noticed.

Sty

A sty is an acute, local, pus-forming infection of the meibomian glands, Moll's glands, or the glands of Zeis. Most often the sty forms on the margin of the eyelid, but may sometimes occur underneath the lid itself. There are, therefore, both external and internal sties. The most frequent causative factor here is the *Staphylococcus aureus* bacterium. The sty normally develops with tenderness of the lid margin and local pain, then later forms a small, round pustule. In general, one could say that a sty is a small boil on the eyelid.

There are a number of homeopathic remedies that have been found useful in treating a sty. Three of the most useful remedies will be presented here.

HOMEOPATHIC TREATMENT
Hepar Sulphuris Calcareum (Hepar Sulph.)
Pulsatilla
Sulphur

Hepar Sulph. is a homeopathic mineral remedy, calcium sulphide. Hepar sulph. is one of the most valuable remedies for treating any pus-forming condition that, like a sty, tends toward suppuration (pus drainage). With Hepar sulph. there will be redness and obvious inflammation of the eyelid and considerable sensitivity to touch or pressure.

Potency and Dosage: Hepar sulph. is an unusual remedy in that it can both prevent suppuration or encourage it, depending on the potency used. *Low potencies* (3x, 6x, or 3c) encourage drainage while *mid-range potencies* (30x, 15c or 30c) absorb the accumulated pus and prevent suppuration and *middle potencies* can act in either direction. If a sty is suspected but not yet formed, a high potency will prevent its formation. If the sty has already formed (pus accumulated) a lower potency will produce drainage.

Pulsatilla is made from a plant commonly called the wind flower. This remedy in homeopathic potency is generally considered *the* most valuable remedy in sties. W. A. Dewey, M.D., considers Pulsatilla "a remedy for styes [without] equal . . . caus[ing] them to abort before pus has formed."[13]

Potency and Dosage: 6x–30x or 30c, one dose every 3 to 4 hours as needed until a noticeable improvement in the condition is seen.

Sulphur is yet another homeopathic remedy, especially for those athletes whose physical makeup creates a tendency toward recurring sties. Sulphur is of special value in all conditions that relapse, as sties often do, and when the Keynote symptoms of localized heat and burning are accompanied by itching. The sensation is made worse from heat. (One of the most common suggestions for treating sties is to place a hot pack on the affected eye. If heat makes the feeling worse, Sulphur will be the first remedy to use.)

Potency and Dosage: 6x–30x or 30c, one dose every 3 to 4 hours as needed until a noticeable improvement in the condition is seen.

Inflammation of the Eyelid: Blepharitis

Blepharitis is a medical term which simply means an acute inflammation of the external margin of the eyelid. In blepharitis there is a thickening of the lid accompanied by redness of the lid margin, and often the formation of scales or crusts and sometimes pinhead-size ulcerations. The cause of this condition is most often bacterial, but sometimes allergic. Under standard (allopathic) medical treatment, blepharitis doesn't respond especially well. Homeopathic treatment, however, often effects a quick healing of the condition.

HOMEOPATHIC TREATMENT
Graphites
Mercurius
Pulsatilla

Graphites is the homeopathically triturated element carbon, sometimes called black lead. A. B. Norton, M.D., considers that "[Graphites] comes nearer being a specific [treatment] in Blepharitis than any other."[14] The following are symptoms:

1. Eyelids are red and swollen.
2. Considerable dryness of the lids is present.
3. Eczema (scales and crusts) form along the lid margins.

Potency and Dosage: Graphites is best used in a low potency (3x or 3c), with one dose given every 2 to 3 hours. The inflammation of the eyelid(s) should resolve itself within 3 days.

Mercurius is a triturated remedy made from mercury (quicksilver). It demonstrates a considerable power over eyelid inflammations of this type, with the following symptoms:

1. The lid(s) is thick, red, and swollen.
2. The discharge from the eye(s) is profuse, acidic, and burning.

Potency and Dosage: Mercurius should not be used in low potencies (below 6x) without a physician's recommendation because of the possibility of mercury poisoning. If symptoms agree, Mercurius may be used in 6x–30x or 30c potencies, one dose every 3 to 4 hours as needed until there is a noticeable improvement of symptoms.

Pulsatilla, the wind flower, shows a special affinity to the eyes. Its Keynote symptoms are:

1. There is considerable itching, burning, and inflammation.
2. Eyelid margins are red and mattery.
3. Eyes may produce a profuse, thick yellow and nonacidic discharge.

Wounds of the Eye

By a wounded eye we refer *only* to a cut to the eyelid itself, and *not* to any injury directly to the eyeball. Any injury to the eyeball requires prompt medical attention.

If the eyelid becomes cut (not an uncommon injury for boxers), the lid should be compressed with a 50/50 solution of CALENDULA in its succus or tincture form and water. Calendula is an outstanding wound treatment made from the fresh (succus) or alcoholic (tincture) extraction of the African marigold plant. Calendula is hemostatic — it slows down, diminishes or stops bleeding. It is also aseptic — works to prevent infection.

In treating the wounded eye, soak a gauze compress or cotton ball in the diluted Calendula solution and apply it directly against the cut. Once bleeding has stopped, Calendula may be reapplied and an adhesive bandage (i.e., a Band-Aid) used to cover the wound.

Concurrent Homeopathic Remedies in Eye Inflammations

The mineral remedy *Ferrum Phosphoricum* (usually called Ferr. phos.) is an excellent adjunctive remedy in any eye inflammation. It is the chemical compound iron phosphate. Ferr. phos. is valuable in any condition where there is burning, redness, and general inflammation. It is *not* suited to any condition where there is a purulent discharge.

Potency and Dosage: Low potencies (3x, 6x or 3c) are most appropriate, and may be repeated frequently. Ferr. phos. is an ideal concurrent remedy when alternated with the specific remedy. It assists in oxygenating the tissues, and oxygen promotes rapid healing.

---

13. W. A. Dewey, M.D., *Practical Homeopathic Therapeutics,* 3d ed. (New Delhi: Jain Publishing Company, Ltd., 1981) p. 150.

14. *Ibid,* p. 155.

CHAPTER SIX

EAR, NOSE, AND THROAT PROBLEMS

Topics Covered

Earache
Otitis Externa (Swimmer's Ear)
Otitis Media (Middle Ear Infection)
Airborne Allergies
Sore Throat and Tonsillitis

Hearing is one of the most complex and delicate of the five physical senses. The ear is composed of three distinct sections, each working in complex interrelationship, and each consisting of structures essential for sound receptivity.

The external ear, also called the *pinna* or *auricle,* is a tough, skin-covered cartilaginous structure that catches and channels sound waves into the ear canal, called the *external auditory meatus.* Lined with a highly specialized skin called the *epithelium,* the ear canal secretes a lubricating wax, *cerumen,* that traps, then expells foreign materials that may enter the outer ear. The eardrum or *tympanic membrane* completely covers and separates the canal from the middle ear.

Beyond the tympanic membrane lies the middle ear, a cubical cavity consisting of the three smallest bones in the body, the *auditory ossicles*—the *malleus, incus,* and *stapes,* also called the hammer, anvil, and stirrup because of their distinctive shapes. Connected to one another and activated by two small muscles, these bones receive sound vibrations from the eardrum and transmit those vibrations into the structures of the inner ear.

The innermost section of the hearing apparatus, the inner ear, consists of a bony labyrinth and a membranous labyrinth, the three *semicircular canals* and a bony *cochlea.* The cochlea, resembling a snail's shell, is divided into chambers which contain a fluid and the *organ of Corti,* lined with fine hairs that respond to and transmit sound wave impulses along the eighth cranial nerve to the brain where hearing is perceived.

This discussion, of course, is not intended to be an exhaustive consideration of the anatomy of the ear. It is intended to be sufficiently instructive to provide the reader with the basic information necessary to understand the complexity of hearing.

It should be noted at this point that homeopathy provides a highly effective treatment for many external and middle ear conditions athletes may encounter.

> ADVISORY WARNING: Due to the delicacy and supreme importance of the sense of hearing, should the best-indicated homeopathic treatment of any ear condition fail to cure the problem within 48 hours, a health care professional must be consulted.

Earache

Simple earache in an athlete is usually caused by exposure to cold or damp, or from a viral cold extending from the sinuses or eustachian tube into the ear. Earache may also result from dental problems. Earache is by far more common among young athletes than in adults.

HOMEOPATHIC TREATMENT
Chamomilla
Ferrum Phosphoricum (Ferr. Phos.)
Plantago Majus Tincture

Chamomilla, made from a trituration of the German chamomile herb, is especially well indicated in earaches in young athletes. However,

Chamomilla is also considered effective in adults, as always, whenever the Keynote symptoms agree:

1. There is ringing in the ears.
2. There is earache with localized soreness.
3. There is a sensation of swelling and heat in the ear.
4. The ear(s) feels congested – stopped up.

Potency and Dosage: Chamomilla is effective in a broad range of potencies from its lowest (3x, 6x and 3c) to mid-range potencies (12x–30x and 12c–30c). Lower potencies require more frequent repetition. 3x and 6x potencies should be repeated every 2 to 3 hours until symptoms subside; midrange potencies every 3 to 4 hours for a maximum of 9 doses.

Ferrum Phosphoricum (Ferr. phos.) is a homeopathic trituration of iron phosphate, a mineral element compound. It is one of the twelve homeopathic mineral elements called "cell" or "tissue" salts.

> "*Ferr. phos.* is the preeminent Biochemic First-Aid [in inflammations of all types]. It enters into the composition of hemoglobin, the red colouring matter of the blood. [Ferr. phos.] takes up oxygen from the air inhaled by the lungs and carries it in the blood stream to all parts of the body. . . . It gives strength and toughness to the . . . blood vessels. . . . *Ferr. phos.* should always be considered, as a supplementary remedy, no matter what other treatment may be indicated by the symptoms.
>
> Congestion, inflammatory pain, high temperature, quickened pulse, all call for more oxygen, and it is *Ferr. phos.* that is the medium through which oxygen is taken up by the blood . . . and carried to the affected area." [15]

Ferr. phos. may be given with considerable advantage at the initial stages of any inflammatory condition, such as earache, and should be given at frequent intervals in the 3x or 6x potency.

Potency and Dosage: A dose of 5 1-grain tablets every 15 to 30 minutes, at the beginning of inflammation. Repeat often throughout a 24-hour period, combining other well-indicated homeopathic medication as needed. Ferr. phos. is best used in its lower, 3x and 6x potencies.

Plantago Majus Tincture, the alcohol and water extract of the plantain, is an excellent and highly effective external medication in simple earache, and most especially when the pain is associated with a toothache. If the earache is associated with a cavity or other dental problem, the underlying cause of the pain must be assessed by a dentist. There are the following symptoms:

1. There is sticking pain in one or both ears.
2. Noise is painful to the patient.
3. Pain seems to run from one ear into the other through the head.
4. Earache symptoms are often associated with a toothache.
5. Pain runs between teeth and ears.

Potency and Dosage: One or two drops of the tincture applied directly to the affected tooth will stop pain temporarily. Applied at no less than room temperature, Plantago majus tincture is effective when placed directly into the ear canal with a loose cotton plug inserted to retain the liquid.

Otitis Externa (Swimmer's Ear)

A localized inflammation of the external auditory meatus, otitis externa is most generally caused by any of several types of bacteria and, rarely, by a fungal infection of the epithelium. Occurring with some frequency during the warm months of summer, the condition among recreational and competitive swimmers is called swimmer's ear.

Swimmer's ear results when contaminated water becomes trapped by debris (cerumen or other foreign matter) and pools within the ear canal. Under these conditions, the epithelial lining becomes macerated and the bacteria or fungus invades the tissue, spreads, and causes an acute infection.

Otitis externa is generally associated with intense itching and pain along and within the auditory meatus. The athlete will sometimes complain of a temporary but distinct hearing loss. In its secondary inflammatory stage, otitis externa may produce swelling of the canal and a purulent, foul discharge from the opening.

As in all health conditions, prevention is better than cure. A number of readily available, over-the-counter medications will help to prevent swimmer's ear. These generally consist of alcohol, boric acid, and benzalkonium chloride.

A very simple preventive remedy frequently used by swim team coaches, and aquatics directors at summer camps, is a one-to-three-part dilution of distilled white vinegar (5% acidity) introduced into the ear in 3- to 4-drop dosages immediately after the swimmer leaves the water. Acetic acid (the acid component of vinegar) alters the pH of the auditory meatus and prevents or at least inhibits the growth of harmful bacteria. The medical profession employs a 0.5% acetic acid solution with a three-times-daily dosage for a week to cure otitis media. Another common treatment for swimmer's ear consists of a combination antibiotic and steroid (Cortisporin), which is available only on a physician's prescription.

If treated in its initial stages with a remedy best indicated by the Keynote symptoms, swimmer's ear yields rapidly to homeopathic treatment. A complete cure can be expected.

HOMEOPATHIC TREATMENT

Aconite
Belladonna
Chamomilla
Pulsatilla
Echinacea Tincture

Swimmer's ear often overlaps the general symptom picture of many of the homeopathic remedies noted above. For that reason, a combination remedy composed of three of the most commonly employed remedies is often best indicated: Aconite, Belladonna, Chamomilla, or ABC. Some homeopathic pharmacies and pharmaceutical manufacturers carry ABC, or it can be specially compounded on request.

To illustrate: A 15-year-old high school competitive swimmer with a history of chronic otitis externa was referred to this writer by his swim coach/father for evaluation. The boy's symptom picture consisted of sharp, needle-like pains and constant itching within the auditory meatus, with the pain developing into a tearing, unbearable constancy. Upon examination with the otoscope, the canal appeared bright red and inflamed. Belladonna, 30c, 5 1-grain tablets taken 4 times daily for 2 days, together with 3 to 4 drops of Echinacea tincture instilled locally into the ear canal, made short work of the infection with complete recovery in 48 hours.

The boy, now 16, takes ABC in 30c combination potency at the earliest stages of infection; he has not had to resort to antibiotic/steroid drugs in over a year.

Aconite responds to the following symptoms:

1. The ear is very sensitive to noise.
2. The external ear is hot, bright red, painful, and swollen.
3. There is earache with the sensation as if a drop of water were trapped inside canal.

The symptoms that indicate using *Belladonna* are:

1. There is tearing pain throughout the auditory meatus.
2. Humming noises are heard.
3. There is considerable sensitivity to loud noises.
4. Pain causes delirium.
5. The eardrum bulges and appears bright red with congested blood vessels upon otoscopic examination.

Using *Chamomilla* is associated with the following symptoms:

1. Ear pains are violent with stitching pains.
2. Pain is worse from warmth.
3. The athlete is restless and fretful.
4. The ear feels stopped up and congested.
5. Swelling and heat causes considerable discomfort.

Pulsatilla aids in the following:

1. The ear is hot, red, and swollen.
2. There are severe, darting and tearing pains, often throbbing in nature, which are most often worse at night.

Potency and Dosage: The potency and dosages for each of the above-listed remedies are the same: best employed in acute otitis externa are the midrange potencies (30x or 30c), although the lower potencies (6x–12x or 3c–6c) are also effective. Midrange potencies should be given every 3 to 4 hours for a maximum of 9 doses; lower potencies every 2 to 3 hours for as long as 24 to 36 hours, as required until a noticeable improvement is established.

As can be readily observed from the Keynote symptoms of Aconite, Belladonna, and Chamomilla, the combination ABC remedy covers the majority of symptoms of otitis externa. Therefore, it would be wise for all swim team coaches, trainers, parents, and athletes to have this remedy available for immediate use.

The alcohol and water extract of the purple cone flower, *Echinacea* tincture is an important and valuable remedy in any localized, external inflammation of the auditory meatus. Echinacea tincture should best be diluted in its tincture form, 9 parts of purified or distilled water to 1 part of the tincture, and instilled directly into the ear canal, in 3- to 4-drop doses, every 2 to 3 hours. As an external application only, Echinacea tincture is best used together with the most appropriate of the other remedies listed.

Otitis Media (Middle Ear Infection)

Normally, acute middle ear infections occur in infants and young children between three months and three years of age. Due to the unique structure of the eustachian tube (its extremely short length and negligible slope in this age group), bacteria travel easily from the naso-pharynx and into the middle ear. Occasionally, however, otitis media will develop in older athletes.

Symptoms of a middle ear infection include sudden and severe earache, elevated fever (101°F at a minimum), and sometimes a loss of hearing acuity, nausea, vomiting, and diarrhea.

A relatively effective means of diagnosis of otitis media is to gently pull downward on the pinna or auricle, and press on the tragus (the small, cartilaginous projection nearest the face). Any resultant pain or general discomfort tends to indicate external ear infection (otitis externa). Pain will not be felt in this procedure in otitis media. Otoscopic examination can readily determine if the tympanic membrane is swollen and red from engorged blood vessels–the generally determining diagnosis of otitis media.

HOMEOPATHIC TREATMENT
Aconite
Belladonna

The two most important Keynote symptoms of **Aconite** in otitis media are physical and mental restlessness. In clinical application, Aconite has proven consistently useful in the initial stages of infection whenever there is a sudden and violent onset of pain accompanied by fever.

Potency and Dosage: The entire potency range of *Aconite* is valuable. The lower potencies (3x–6x or 3c) are given every 2 to 3 hours and repeated for as long as 48 hours, or until there is noticeable improvement in symptoms. The mid-range potencies (30x and 30c) work more rapidly. Dosage for mid-range potencies is every 3 to 4 hours for a maximum of 9 doses.

Belladonna most often covers the common Keynote symptoms of otitis media. The eardrum upon otoscopic examination will be bright red and congested, bulging outward. The athlete experiences throbbing, beating, or tearing pains deep within the ear.

Potency and Dosage: Same as for Aconite.

Airborne Allergies

A common complaint among athletes at various times of the sporting season is allergy: the sniffling, sneezing, watery, sometimes blood-shot eyes, produced by airborne pollens or mold spores.

The severity of overall symptoms varies greatly from person to person, from mild and annoying and moderate, to severe and debilitating. As most allergy sufferers know, over-the-counter and prescription antihistamines often produce a sedating effect. Concentration then becomes difficult.

Certainly, credit must be granted the orthodox medical profession in its recent development of antihistamine-like drugs that do not penetrate the blood/brain barrier of the central nervous system and, in the vast majority of patients, produce no sedating effects.

Homeopathic treatment, however, frequently produces long-term, and often permanent relief from symptoms. And, unlike most pharmaceutical products, homeopathic remedies produce none of the common side effects of antihistamines. Permanent, curative treatment for airborne allergies is the province of the trained homeopathic health care professional. Athletes may, however, benefit greatly from the symptomatic treatment of acute allergic conditions.

The symptomatic treatment of airborne allergies lessens or temporarily removes symptoms. Symptomatic treatment is not curative.

The most direct and simplified approach to a seasonal airborne allergy is to employ a suitable combination remedy. These proprietary combinations are readily available from homeopathic pharmacies and pharmaceutical manufacturers. They generally work exceedingly well.

Through its *Materia Medica,* homeopathy does offer many single remedies that effectively treat allergic symptoms, so the following list should not be considered exhaustive.

The most significant advantage homeopathic treatment can offer the majority of hayfever sufferers over its allopathic counterpart is painless and permanent desensitization.

Annually, thousands of hayfever and allergy sufferers flock into allopathic allergy clinics, first, to undergo a series of skin patch testing to determine the specific substance(s) they are allergic to, and second, to submit to a lengthy series of weekly or twice-weekly injections. This method, called *isotherapy,* employs minute amounts of the allergens to which the person is allergic—house dust, cat hair, molds, pollens, even food substances—to establish desensitization. Not only is the procedure lengthy, lasting a year or longer, but uncomfortable, and very expensive.

Although they may not willingly acknowledge it, allergists using isotherapy are employing a form of homeopathy. True homeopathic treatment of allergies may not employ the specific substance to which a person is sensitive, but it does employ a substance which, in crude form, would produce a very similar symptom picture to that which the person is experiencing. Homeopathy, however, also employs isotherapy.

Based upon a complete health history and a thorough analysis of the patient's Keynote symptoms, a homeopathic or naturopathic physician can locate and prescribe *the* single isotherapeutic substance in homeopathic potency that most fits the overall allergic symptoms.

As is true in allopathic practice, homeopathic desensitization requires great care in effective prescribing, and, usually, a two- to three-year course of treatment, before a long-term remission of symptoms can be achieved. But the results are very often well worth the time required, and the advantages are numerous: there is no pain through hypodermic injections; there are no continuous office visits; and homeopathically prepared remedies are cheap.

Allergy management is tricky at best. Lay persons should not expect to desensitize themselves. However, using classical homeopathy, once the most similar single remedy is found, the lay prescriber can, by taking that remedy at least six weeks prior to the usual onset of seasonal symptoms, produce a significant seasonal desensitization.

The effectiveness of the homeopathic approach to allergy management has been well documented over decades of clinical practice. Its safety and positive results are well known in homeopathy, naturopathy, and holistic health care.

HOMEOPATHIC TREATMENT
Allium Cepa
Ambrosia
Arsenicum Album (Arsenicum Alb.)
Euphrasia
Naphthaline
Pothos Foetida
Sabadilla

Always remember, when selecting a single remedy, to *match the symptoms of the remedy with the overall symptoms you are experiencing.* Employ the homeopathic "three-legged stool." This is a means for selecting the remedy the most similar to the complaint, and is as old as homeopathy itself. You cannot balance on a two-legged stool, but put three legs under it, and it is solid. In homeopathic prescribing, find three key or major symptoms under a single remedy that most match your prominent symptoms and, nine times out of ten, you will have found the correct remedy for your particular symptom pattern.

Allium Cepa, frequently called upon when the hayfever sufferer does not sneeze, is made from the common red onion. Anyone who has sliced an onion well knows this pungent vegetable's effects! In homeopathy, the symptoms a substance can produce, it can also cure. Allium is one of homeopathy's most effective and often-called-on remedies for hayfever when the Keynote symptoms agree:

1. There is acid, burning discharge from the nose.
2. The nose becomes red and sore.
3. The eyes are red and water profusely, but the discharge is bland and nonirritating.
4. The eyelids are sore and burn.

Ambrosia is not the "nectar of the gods" of Greek mythology to hayfever sufferers, but the Latin botanical name for the common ragweed, which brings hayfever symptoms to millions. Ambrosia's Keynote symptoms are:

1. There is much watering from the eyes with intolerable itching of the eyelids.
2. The nose and head feel stuffed up.
3. There is sneezing with watery discharge from the nose.

Arsenicum Alb. is the remedy made from the compound arsenic trioxide, and is frequently found to be very useful in treating hayfever symptoms. In its homeopathic form, it is perfectly safe. It should not be used below the 6x or 3c potency. Arsenicum's Keynote symptoms are:

1. There is a thin, watery discharge from the nose; the discharge burns the upper lip.
2. The nose is stuffed up; although there is much sneezing, it brings no relief.
3. All symptoms are worse in the open air and better indoors.

Euphrasia is a wonderful remedy in hayfever in which eye symptoms predominate. In fact, the common name of this herb is eyebright. Euphrasia's Keynote symptoms include:

1. The nose runs profusely, especially in the morning.
2. The eyes water constantly, burn, and discharge a yellow, sticky matter.
3. The eyelids burn and swell.
4. All symptoms are worse in the evening and indoors.

Euphrasia can be made into a soothing eyewash by adding 5 drops of the tincture to a half-cup of pure, distilled water, the mixture placed in an eye cup, or instilled with an eyedropper. The tincture, which has a high concentration of alcohol, must NEVER be placed directly into the eyes. Euphrasia Eye Lotion is readily available in Britain.

Naphthaline is a coal tar compound and is often found in combination with other remedies. Alone, Naphthaline's Keynote symptoms are:

1. There is much sneezing.
2. The eyes are inflamed and painful, and burn.
3. The eyelids are often swollen.
4. The head feels hot.

Pothos Foetida is made from the common skunk cabbage and its Keynote symptoms include:

1. Allergic symptoms are made worse from breathing dust.
2. Sneezing is accompanied by a pain in the throat.
3. There is difficult breathing with accompanying pain(s) in the chest.

Sabadilla is made from the cevadilla seed and produces very typical hayfever symptoms when accompanied by pains in the front of the head. Sabadilla's Keynote symptoms are:

1. There is spasmodic sneezing accompanied by a runny nose.
2. The eyes are red and watery, and burn.
3. All symptoms are most often accompanied by frontal head pains.

Sore Throat and Tonsillitis

Although most athletes, as well as the general sporting public, are inclined to consider a sore throat the same as tonsillitis, the two diseases are not the same.

The sore throat is best termed *pharyngitis,* an acute inflammation of the pharynx that produces pain upon swallowing. Pharyngitis is most often the result of a viral infection. Although not as common, it may be, as well, the result of bacterial infection: streptococcus or (more rarely) staphylococcus or other bacteria.

Tonsillitis is an inflammation of the tonsils themselves. Tonsillitis produces a severe pain upon swallowing. The pain often shoots into the ears and is accompanied by a fever (102°–103°F). There is moderate to severe tiredness, and a headache. Though tonsillitis is caused by several infective agents, probably 85% of it is viral in origin, the remaining 15% the result of streptococcal ("Strep Throat") infection or other bacteria.

Should a simple sore throat be treated by antibiotics? Even the medical profession does not agree. Many physicians today recommend as the primary therapy, rest, aspirin for fever, and hydrogen peroxide gargles. Antibiotics are reserved for the more serious bacterial infections, but are not, of course, effective against the virus. (NOTE: *Aspirin is best not taken by anyone under age 18 due to its association with the development of Reye's Syndrome following viral infections).*

In the treatment of pharyngitis and tonsillitis homeopathy clearly demonstrates its rapid, curative power. Using either a well-selected single remedy by its overall Keynote symptoms, or a combination remedy, the athlete may expect a marked improvement or complete cure of both conditions in as little as 24 hours, but more commonly in 36–48 hours.

HOMEOPATHIC TREATMENT
Aconite
Apis Melifica (Apis Mel.)

Belladonna
Hepar Sulphuris Calcareum
Lachesis
Lycopodium
Phytolacca Decandra

Aconite is most effective at the initial stage of throat symptoms, and generally ineffective after a sore throat is entrenched. It is an outstanding remedy. The Keynote symptoms are:

1. The throat is red and dry.
2. The patient complains of a constricted feeling in the throat.
3. The patient has difficulty upon swallowing and speaking.
4. The throat is red, but *not* bright red or glossy.
5. The patient may complain of a burning or pricking sensation in the throat.

An important Aconite modality as it relates to sore throats is that both hot and cold liquids disagree.

Potency and Dosage: Aconite works effectively in a broad range of potencies from low (6x or 3c) to the midrange (12x–30x or 30c) potencies. Lower potencies require more frequent repetition over a longer time: 1 dose every 2 to 3 hours for 24 to 48 hours, or until symptoms abate. Midrange potencies should be administered every 3 to 4 hours for a maximum of 9 doses, as required.

Apis Mel. is one of the major remedies in the homeopathic *Materia Medica* in all types of sore throats, regardless of cause, whenever its Keynote symptoms agree:

1. The throat is swollen, both inside and outside.
2. There are stinging pains.
3. There is a sensation of constriction in the throat.
4. The throat and/or tonsils are fiery red, puffy.
5. The *uvula* (the bag-shaped organ at the back of the throat) is often swollen and fiery red.

6. The throat is worse from hot liquids, from pressure and touch, and better from cold liquids.
7. The throat often feels as if a fishbone were caught in it.

Potency and Dosage: The same as for Aconite.

Belladonna is made from the deadly nightshade plant, and demonstrates the following Keynote symptoms:

1. The throat is dry, angry red and glossy (shiny).
2. The throat feels greatly constricted, with much difficulty on swallowing.
3. The tonsils may or may not be swollen.
4. The throat is worse on the right side; from swallowing any liquid, and from pressure and touch.

The strongest Keynote symptom of the Belladonna throat is its bright, shiny-red appearance.

Potency and Dosage: The same as for Aconite.

Hepar Sulph. is a mineral compound originally developed by the founder of modern homeopathy, Samuel Hahnemann, M.D. Its Keynote symptoms are:

1. The throat feels as if a plug or splinter were stuck in it.
2. Sharp, needle-like pains run from the throat into the ear upon swallowing.
3. There is much "hawking" as the patient attempts to clear the throat of clinging mucus.
4. The tonsils may appear ulcerated or abscessed.
5. Pain is worse from cold liquids; better from warm liquids and after eating.

Potency and Dosage: The same as for Aconite.

Lachesis is one of the most powerful homeopathic remedies triturated from the venom of the surucucu snake. In its homeopathic microdiluted state, it retains an amazing curative power while losing its poison quality. The Keynote symptoms are:

1. The throat is exceptionally dry.
2. There is intense swelling of both the inside and outside of the throat.
3. The slightest touch is painful.
4. Pain runs from the throat to the ear(s).
5. The throat is *severely* painful with enlarged, dark-colored, or purplish tonsils.
6. Pain is worse on the left side, on swallowing liquids, greatly aggravated by hot drinks; better from warm local applications to the neck.

Potency and Dosage: The same as for Aconite.

Lycopodium is made from the trituration of the club moss plant spores. It is a key ally in the treatment of pharyngitis and tonsillitis, its Keynote symptoms well targeted.

1. Throat pain always begins on the right side, remains on the right, or moves from the right side to the left.
2. Throat symptoms generally develop from 4:00 to 8:00 PM.
3. The throat is dry.
4. The patient is totally without thirst.
5. The throat is inflamed, accompanied by sharp, needle-like pains upon swallowing.
6. In advanced inflammation, food or liquids are often regurgitated through the nose.
7. Pain is worse from cold drinks; better from warm liquids.

Potency and Dosage: The same as for Aconite.

Phytolacca Decandra has the following Keynote symptoms:

1. The throat is dark red to bluish in color.
2. The root, or base, of the tongue is painful.

3. The soft palate (fleshy portion behind the hard roof of the mouth) is sore.

4. Tonsils may be swollen, dark red or bluish.

5. Pain shoots into the ears upon swallowing.

6. The throat feels hot with a burning sensation.

7. An advanced sore throat shows ulcerated tonsils with gray-white spots and thick, yellow mucus at the back of the throat and/or on the tonsils.

Potency and Dosage: The same as for Aconite.

Commonly available combination remedies in homeopathic potency, in either tablet or liquid form, are available from homeopathic pharmacies and pharmaceutical manufacturers. These combinations make the selection of the most appropriate remedy simple and combine a majority of the most commonly required single remedies.

---

15. *The Biochemic Handbook* (St. Louis, MO: Formur, Inc., 1973) p. 14.

CHAPTER SEVEN

COMMON INJURIES

Topics Covered

Sprains
Tennis Elbow and Golfer's Elbow
Old Sprains
Bruises
Bone Bruises
Dislocations
Fractures

Sprains

A sprain is usually a painful injury resulting from damage to ligaments, the tough, fibrous, elastic connective tissues surrounding joints. The most common sites of sprains in sporting injuries are the ankles, wrists, and thumbs. In a sprain, the ligaments are stretched and, in severe sprains, actually torn away from the joint.

Sprains, by far the most common sports injury of the lower extremities, are classified by severity: *first, second,* and *third* degree. For a first degree sprain, pain, tenderness, and swelling surround the joint. Swelling is minimal, though, with little or no skin discoloration from the hemorrhage of blood into surrounding tissues. For a second degree sprain, in addition to local tenderness, which is more pronounced and intense, there is greater swelling, some discoloration of the surrounding skin, and some limitation of motion of the joint. The more intense tenderness and restriction of motion is the Keynote symptom in a second degree sprain. For a third degree sprain, in addition to the symptoms noted above, there is instability of the joint, a feeling in the injured joint as if it were giving way.

First and second degree sprains generally require only symptomatic treatment. A sprain of the third degree, however, because of the difficulty in diagnosis, requires evaluation and treatment by a specialist, a sports orthopedist.

In treating both first and second degree sprains, think A.R.I.C.E.H.

A = Anti-inflammatory medication
R = Rest
I = Ice
C = Compression
E = Elevation
H = Heat

A.R.I.C.E.H. is the traditional form of medical and first-aid treatment for sprains. *A* is anti-inflammatory. The anti-inflammatory medications normally include aspirin (nonaspirin medications such as Tylenol and other acetaminophen products do not have anti-inflammatory properties), and the nonsteroidal drugs such as Advil, Nuprin, and the prescription pharmaceuticals Motrin and Naprosin. Homeopathic medicine does not employ anti-inflammatory drugs and does not recommend their use. *R* stands for rest. The injured part is kept motionless. For upper extremity injuries, a sling may be required for up to three days. *I* is ice. An ice pack or chemical cold pack is applied directly over the injured joint and surrounding tissues for 10 minutes every hour. Depending on the severity of the sprain this cold treatment may need to be continued for 24 to 48 hours. *C* is for compression. Compressing the tissues near the site of the injury permits swelling to be reduced. Swelling in any sprain is caused by blood and intercellular fluids leaking from damaged tissues. Compression is accomplished by applying an elastic bandage on, and immediately above and below, the site of injury. An elastic wrap does provide some stability to the injury and helps limit motion. The wrap should not be applied too tightly. If numbness or a change in skin color should occur around the bandage, it is too tight and is disturbing the circulation. If this occurs, remove the bandage and rewrap it more loosely. *E* stands for elevation. Raising the injured limb above heart level permits gravity to assist in draining any excess fluids and thereby reduces swelling and inflammation. *H* stands for heat. Most sports physicians and trainers recommend that, following 24 hours or less of cold treatment, heat be applied. Use a heating pad or infrared lamp. Heat permits dilation of the blood vessels, which assists in the reduction of inflammation and the elimination of metabolic (toxic) wastes.

Homeopathic approaches to sprains of the first and second degree are very similar to those recommended above. Homeopathic treatment rewrites the formula as H.R.I.C.E.H. The first *H* stands for homeopathic remedy.

In addition to the simple symptomatic first-aid treatment outlined above, homeopathic therapies are meant to provide rapid elimination of pain, reduced swelling, and fast recovery.

HOMEOPATHIC TREATMENT
Arnica Montana
Bryonia
Rhus Toxicodendron (Rhus Tox.)
Ruta Graveolens (Ruta Grav.)

Arnica (Arnica montana) should be considered *first* in all cases of physical injury and is often considered *the* preeminent remedy in first and second degree sprains. Arnica works quickly to repair damaged blood vessels, to reduce swelling at the site of the injury, and to eliminate pain. Arnica is not, however, an analgesic. It has no pain-relieving properties of its own. The considerable and rapid reduction or elimination of pain following Arnica is probably due to its ability to greatly reduce swelling in most injuries.

Potency and Dosage: 6x–30x or 30c, 1 dose every 30 minutes for 3 to 4 doses, then 1 dose 3 times a day as needed for pain and swelling.

Bryonia is the homeopathic remedy made from the herb wild hops. Bryonia is prescribed on the modality, "all movement makes the injury worse." In Bryonia, any movement of the injured part is worse and all movement increases the discomfort.

To illustrate: A 16-year-old swim team member this writer treated jammed his thumb into the pool wall during a practice heat. The thumb was swollen, red, extremely tender, and impossible to move without pain. His coach applied a cold pack and recommended elevation. A few hours later, I saw the boy. Arnica 30c was given for the pain and swelling. Based upon the modality, "all movement difficult and painful," Bryonia 30c was prescribed, to be taken after the initial doses of Arnica.

The boy's injury was a second degree sprain and severe enough to have required 14 to 21 days of support before complete healing occurred. However, on a follow-up visit three days after the injury, swelling had diminished to nearly normal, pain and tenderness had totally subsided, and he enjoyed a nearly complete free range of movement in the thumb. In the following few days there was no sign of injury whatsoever. Under standard medical practice this second degree sprain should have taken up to seven times longer to heal.

Potency and Dosage: 6x–30x or 30c, 1 dose every 30 minutes for 3 to 4 doses, then 1 dose 3 times a day as needed until noticeable improvement is established.

Rhus Tox. is one of the most common homeopathic medicines used in the treatment of sprains. However, in order for Rhus tox. to function effectively, its Keynote symptoms must agree.

An extract and trituration of poison ivy, in its pure, undiluted form Rhus tox. produces the same symptoms commonly found in sprains: painful tenderness and stiffness around joints, in the ligaments and tendons. This is why homeopaths so often think of Rhus tox. as being almost specific to all joint injuries. The Keynote symptom of Rhus tox. is that the injury "feels better from movement." Notice that this symptom is the exact *opposite* of Bryonia.

Potency and Dosage: 6x–30x or 30c, 1 dose every 30 minutes for 3 to 4 doses, then 1 dose 3 to 4 times a day as needed until noticeable improvement is established.

Ruta Grav. (Ruta graveolens) is a deep-acting homeopathic medicine, demonstrating a strong affinity to injuries of the ligaments and tendons, especially where the ligaments and tendons have been torn or stretched. Ruta grav. is not a remedy to consider at the outset of the injury, which other, more symptom-specific remedies would best cover. Ruta grav.

follows Rhus tox. well, and is best employed following a reduction in swelling and pain, or following any of the best-suggested remedies if they have failed to significantly improve the condition within a reasonable time.

The Keynote symptom of Ruta grav. is "injury is neither definitely worse by motion nor significantly improved by continued movement."

Potency and Dosage: 6x–30x or 30c, 1 dose every 30 minutes for 3 to 4 doses, then 1 dose 3 to 4 times daily as required until noticeable improvement is established.

Tennis Elbow and Golfer's Elbow

Tennis elbow in medical terminology is called *lateral epicondylitis* because localized inflammation occurs at the origin of the supinator muscles of the lateral epicondyle region. The condition, not uncommon in professional players as well as beginners and weekend warriors, is usually caused by excessive strain of the muscles of the forearm where they attach below the elbow, but can be caused by strain, tearing, and local inflammation of the tendons on the outside of the elbow.

Two types of tennis elbow are recognized, *forehand tennis elbow* and *backhand tennis elbow*. *FTE* is especially common in professional players, and the pain is felt in the muscles on the inner aspect of the elbow. *BTE* is generally a condition of nonprofessionals, caused by an incorrect backhand stroke, with pain felt at the outside of the elbow.

Tennis elbow is not an injury limited to tennis players only. Cross-country skiers, baseball and softball players, even bowlers and mechanics can develop this condition. Even homemakers can develop the symptoms of tennis elbow from opening too many well-stuck jar lids. Any time stresses are placed on the elbow or at the wrist, where motion places stress on the inner or outer aspects of the forearm muscles, tennis elbow can result.

Similar to tennis elbow in general symptom patterns, golfer's elbow, or *medial epicondylitis*, is an inflammation of the flexor and pronator muscles at their origin on the humerus, the bone of the upper arm. Perhaps the only difference in symptomatology between golfer's elbow and tennis elbow is an occasional (though not common) complaint of paresthesia—itching, tingling, or pricking sensations along the ulnar nerve along the inner aspect of the upper and lower arm.

In terms of standard treatment, only rest (a cessation of play), muscle-strengthening exercises, and qualified coaching in the proper racket and club techniques are currently recognized.

Homeopathy adds an additional component to standard approaches while recognizing rest, exercise, and proper coaching as vital ingredients in preventing recurrence of the injury.

HOMEOPATHIC TREATMENT
Arnica Montana
Ruta Graveolens (Ruta Grav.)

Arnica is the first remedy to consider in all muscle-related injuries. It produces a rapid soothing and healing effect on muscle fibers.

Potency and Dosage: 6x–30x or 30c potencies are especially effective. Repeat 1 dose every 30 minutes for 3 to 4 doses at the outset of the injury, then proceed with Ruta grav. as indicated below.

Ruta Grav. is very nearly specific to the symptomatic complaints of tennis and golfer's elbow. A deep-acting remedy, it is highly beneficial when taken internally in homeopathic potency following several initial doses of Arnica, and in its ointment form applied locally.

Potency and Dosage: 6x–30x or 30c, 1 dose 3 to 4 times daily for several days until symptoms considerably abate. Rest from the aggravation that produced the injury initially will be required.

Old Sprains

It is not an uncommon occurrence for athletes who have sustained several or especially severe sprains to experience a continued weakness around the damaged joint. Such a condition can be severely debilitating and force all but the most determined athlete from further participation in play.

These athletes experience a continued discomfort and frequently a permanent, nagging weakness in the joint. The affected joint is easily re-injured.

Mountain hikers and backpackers are certainly athletes. They may not be thin-clads racing around a track, or padded and helmeted American football players. However, carrying thirty- and forty-pound backpacks loaded with food, cooking and camping gear, they are indeed members of the sporting elite.

The young man who came to see me did not appear especially athletic. He was overweight and slow-moving, and yet, with a great deal of stamina. Nothing in his health history indicated that he could not participate well in mountain hiking, his favorite (and only) sport.

He was only 21, but had experienced frequent first and second degree sprains of both ankles since he'd been 14. When he was 19 he had fractured his right ankle so severely that surgical intervention was required. Yet he continued his strenuous outdoor activities. His right ankle, especially, was in constant pain and prone to reinjury. His left ankle was weak as well.

Calc. carb. in a homeopathic 30c potency was prescribed, taken once a week until some improvement became apparent. Following several doses of the remedy, he again twisted his right ankle. A painful and debilitating second degree sprain might have been expected. However, not only did this not occur, but the old injury was not aggravated. And as time passed, there appeared to be no apparent sign of the former weakness in either ankle. There was also a possibility that the ankles would return to near-normal condition.

HOMEOPATHIC TREATMENT
Calcium Carbonate (Calc. Carb.)

Calc. Carb. (homeopathic calcium carbonate) is the remedy of choice in repeated sprains and in those injuries to joints producing continued aggravation. Used as directed, Calc. carb. may greatly assist the weakened joint to a complete and permanent recovery.

Potency and Dosage: Calc. carb. should not be taken above the 30c potency or repeated for more than 1 dose per week. Calc. carb. is an especially deep-acting drug of a constitutional nature and does not bear too-frequent repetition.

Bruises

A bruise, or *contusion,* is any injury produced by the impact of a hard object against the soft tissue structures of the body. In a bruise, the tissues beneath the skin's surface are damaged, and small, peripheral vessels ruptured, with blood and other cellular fluids leaking into the surrounding tissues. The characteristic black-and-blue discoloration of the bruise is the sign of this leakage of blood and other fluids.

The pain of a bruise is usually mild to moderate, and the accompanying swelling moderate to severe.

HOMEOPATHIC TREATMENT
Arnica Montana
Bellis Perennis
Hamamelis

Arnica is an excellent remedy to consider first in all cases of contusions. Although it has no analgesic action of its own, it offers remarkably rapid pain relief. For centuries the Arnica herb, in nonhomeopathic potency, has been chewed to good effect by European mountain climbers and hikers whenever they experience a fall. In its homeopathic triturated potencies, Arnica relieves the lame, sore, stiff, bruised feeling from muscle strains, and simple overexertion.

Potency and Dosage: Any potency of Arnica is useful. The preferred potencies are 6x–30x or 6c–30c. The lower potencies (6x and 6c) are slower acting and require longer repetition. In general first-aid treatment for athletic bruises, Arnica in 30x or 30c potency, 1 dose every half hour to one hour for several doses until a noticeable improvement occurs, is recommended.

Bellis Perennis, a homeopathic preparation made from the common daisy, acts directly on muscle tissues and the fibers of the subcutaneous blood vessels. Bellis follows the administration of Arnica well and the two remedies are totally compatible. Under Bellis, which is well indicated in deep-tissue injuries, healing is rapid.

Potency and Dosage: Bellis perennis is best used in its lower potencies (3x, 6x, or 3c). Single dosages should be repeated frequently until a noticeable improvement occurs.

Other bruise-specific remedies such as **Ruta graveolens** and **Symphytum** will be discussed below. However, bruises of the breast(s) of female athletes respond well to **Conium**. **Hamamelis,** a trituration of witch hazel, follows Arnica well, on those rare occasions when it fails to "hold" or to be effective.

Potency and Dosage: 6x–30x or 30c potencies are advised, administered as prescribed for Arnica.

Bone Bruises

Bone (periosteal) bruises are frequent occurrences in athletic competition. They are most common in football, hockey, and soccer players.

A bone bruise is an injury to the periosteum, the thin sheath covering of the skeletal system. Periosteal injuries are often painful, and indicated by localized tenderness at the site of the injury, swelling, and skin discoloration.

HOMEOPATHIC TREATMENT
Ruta Graveolens
Symphytum

Ruta Graveolens, discussed in some depth under tennis and golfer's elbow injuries, is a truly outstanding remedy in all periosteal bruises.

Symphytum, homeopathic comfrey, is concomitant and complementary to Ruta grav. in periosteal injuries. Should Ruta not take effect within 24 hours, Symphytum, with its deeper-acting properties, is the next step.

Potency and Dosage: Both Ruta and Symphytum are available in tablet and ointment preparations from homeopathic pharmacies. All potencies of both remedies are effective, with the lower potencies to be taken over longer periods. To assist in healing, the ointment (called *cerates* in homeopathy) may be applied externally, several times daily.

Dislocations

ADVISORY WARNING: Any dislocation of a major joint is a serious injury and requires the attention of a physician to relocate the displaced joint.

In a dislocation, ligaments (which bind the joints together) and tendons (which attach muscles to bones), nerves and blood vessels may all be involved. Dislocations should always be treated as fractures; the affected joint should be immobilized, placed in a sling, and strapped firmly to the body.

Most dislocations occur to the shoulder. However, they may occur to any other joint: knees, elbows, fingers, thumbs, jaw, hip, or ankle. The Keynote symptoms of a dislocation are:

1. There is rapid swelling.
2. There is moderate to severe pain.
3. There is obvious deformity of the affected body part.

In dislocation injuries, the bone end pulls away from its joint. The accompanying pain may be excruciating and shock a strong possibility.

HOMEOPATHIC TREATMENT
Arnica Montana
Ruta Graveolens
Bryonia

If possible before, during, or immediately following standard first-aid treatment, give **Arnica** in mid- or high-range potencies to forestall shock, and to assist in reducing blood vessel trauma. Once the affected joint has been relocated by a physician, **Ruta grav.** (6x–30x or 30c) will assist in relieving the associated trauma.

Should the site of a dislocation become swollen following relocation, and worse on the slightest movement, **Bryonia** (6x–30x or 30c) should be administered with Arnica concomitantly, as pain develops.

Fractures

Any fracture or suspected fracture requires the practiced skill of a physician to reduce the break. Some fractures resulting from athletic injuries will require surgical repair.

The athlete and coach should certainly remember that the symptoms of a fracture can be similar to those of a severe second or third degree sprain, with their characteristic and pronounced swelling and tenderness. In sprains, the pain is normally distributed over a wider area than in a fracture, but this is not always a definitive symptom. Keynote symptoms of fracture are:

1. There is swelling at the site of the injury.
2. There is localized pain upon the least movement or touch or pressure.
3. There is limitation in the normal range of motion, with pain.
4. There may be deformity of the injured limb.

HOMEOPATHIC TREATMENT
Arnica Montana
Symphytum Officinale

In any suspected, or proven, fracture, look for shock, which may often accompany even slight injuries. The major symptoms of shock are:

1. The skin is pale, ashen gray, or white.
2. There is profuse sweating.
3. The pupils of the eyes are fixed (unmoving) and dilated (wide open).
4. The victim is lethargic, disoriented, or unconscious.

Administer *Arnica* in a mid-range to high potency (30x–200x or 30c–200c) immediately. Given immediately following injury, Arnica has been proven to prevent shock or to forestall its onset.

Following the reduction of the fracture, homeopathic *Symphytum* in a low potency (3x, 6x, or 3c) has been demonstrated to assist in the formation of new bone. There is no danger, and considerable benefit, to be derived from this post-fracture treatment.

CHAPTER EIGHT

HEAT-STRESS ILLNESS

Topics Covered

Heatstroke
Heat Exhaustion
Heat Cramps

Athletes in Britain and in other cool climates generally have more of a problem with cold than with heat, but it is still vital to drink plenty of fluids,[16] and particularly important to be aware of the additional risks when competing in a hot climate. The *Position Statement on the Prevention of Heat Injuries During Distance Running* of the American College of Sports Medicine is good advice in such conditions:

1. Distance races greater than 16 kilometers or 10 miles should *not* be conducted when the wet bulb temperature wind thermometer exceeds 28°C/82.4°F.

2. During the periods of the year when the daylight dry bulb temperature exceeds 27°C/80°F distance races should be conducted before 9:00 A.M. or after 4:00 P.M.

3. It is the responsibility of the race sponsors to provide fluids that contain a small amount of sugar (less than 2.5 grams glucose per 100 ml. of water) and electrolytes (less than 10 mEq sodium and 5 mEq potassium per liter of solution).

4. Runners should be encouraged to ingest fluids frequently during competition and to consume two glasses of fluid 10 to 15 minutes before competitions.

5. Rules prohibiting the administration of fluids during the first 10 kilometers (6.2 miles) of a marathon race should be amended to permit fluid ingestion at frequent intervals along the race course. In light of the high sweat rates and body temperatures during distance running in the heat, race sponsors should provide water stations at 3 to 4 kilometer (2 to 2.5 mile) intervals for all races of 16 kilometers (10 miles) or more.

6. To avoid heat injury, runners should know its early warning symptoms. As soon as they recognize those symptoms they must cease running and obtain treatment. Early warning symptoms include piloerection on chest and upper arms, chilling throbbing pressure in head, unsteadiness, nausea, and dry skin.

7. Race sponsors should have made prior arrangements with medical personnel for the care of heat injury cases. Responsible and informed personnel should supervise each feeding station. Organizational personnel should reserve the right to stop runners who exhibit clear signs of heatstroke or heat exhaustion.

There exist an extraordinary number of fallacies, myths, and downright dangerous bits of nonsense concerning hot weather sporting competition among athletes. The following section will attempt to dispel some of those falsehoods and prevent heat-stress illness.

1. Athletes must precondition for hot weather competition: Competition in hot weather and high humidity requires additional training to acclimatize the body to new stress. Evaporation of moisture from the body during competition is greater under hot weather conditions than in cool. Cardiac stress is greater in warm weather and under conditions of high humidity.

2. Athletes must train early for hot weather and high humidity competition: Because the athlete perspires far more heavily during hot

weather, the body must be adjusted to these conditions. Before attempting any competition, the athlete should prepare by heavy perspiration training methods at least two weeks in advance of the competition. This extra training should be accomplished by wearing sweats. Many male athletes prefer to train shirtless. Shirtless training, however, does not permit the body to perspire as freely as when the chest and extremities are well covered. Adequate covering permits the body to perspire freely and adjust its internal thermic regulating mechanisms.

3. Athletes must expect lower performance under hot weather conditions: Heat and accompanying high humidity reduce athletic performance, strength, and overall endurance. These two factors, working in tandem, greatly reduce overall performance. The athlete must learn to pace himself or herself during warm weather competition.

4. Athletes must not take salt tablets: As will be explained, athletes generally do not lose large quantities of sodium (salt) during sporting competition. More fluid than salt is lost during sporting activities, and with the decrease in body-fluid volume, what sodium *is* contained in the body is greatly "compressed" and elevated. Such sodium concentrations can lead to serious health problems. Athletes should learn to leave both salt tablets and the salt shaker alone.

5. Athletes must replace minerals: The most common mineral element lost during hot weather sporting is *potassium*. Potassium is available in high concentrations in fruits, vegetables, and their juices. Such juices and foods should become a staple dietary item for any athlete during hot weather competition.

6. Athletes must drink plenty of fluids: An old and very dangerous myth still considered true by many athletes is that they will become waterlogged if they drink fluids prior to competition. The greatest danger an athlete faces during hot weather activity is the excessive loss of body fluids. Well-trained and accomplished athletes drink plenty of fluids—*often*. And, the best drink is still pure water.

7. Athletes should not use commercially prepared drinks for fluid replacement: Available under many brand names, commercially prepared drinks have flooded the sporting market in recent years. These drinks are too highly concentrated to be of positive benefit to the athlete. If they must be drunk, most sports medicine practitioners

recommend that the powdered or already-prepared liquid drinks be diluted with water to 25% to 50% of normal strength.

Carbonated beverages also contain very high concentrations of sugar and athletes should avoid them. Drink plain water, or fruit and vegetable juices that contain potassium.

8. Athletes should drink cold fluids during competition: Recent medical sports research has clearly demonstrated that cold drinks are more rapidly absorbed by the body than cool or warm drinks. And, a common myth has been displaced by the research: Athletes do not experience cramping from ingesting cold drinks in hot weather.

9. Athletes must wear sufficient clothing during hot weather activity: The athlete competing in hot and humid weather requires sufficient body covering to protect himself or herself from the ravaging effects of the sun, but not so much clothing as to restrict perspiration. One of the greatest mistakes the "weekend warrior" can make is to wear nonporous plastic, rubber, or nylon sweats in an abortive attempt to lose weight.

Athletes should always wear some form of upper body covering. Light-weight and light-colored materials are best. They permit free perspiration (which cools the body) and prevent the discomforts and damaging effects of sunburn.

10. Athletes must keep realistic expectations of performance levels: With any increase in heat and humidity, athletic performance drops. This is natural and is always expected by well-trained competitors. Proper prior preparation and sensible training methods go hand in hand in hot weather sporting. Realize that performance peaks lower in hot weather, and many problems with heat-related stress factors will be avoided.

Heat stress may demonstrate itself in one of four symptomologies or syndromes:

1. *Heat Stroke* (rapid increase in body temperature to 105°F–110°F)
2. *Heat Fatigue* (a dysfunction of the muscles; muscle weakness)
3. *Heat Exhaustion* (general weakness, heavy sweating, dizziness and light-headedness without a significant increase in body temperature)
4. *Heat Cramps* (a symptom of sodium loss and/or shifts in the electrolyte balance)

Heatstroke

Heatstroke, also termed sunstroke and thermic fever, is a genuine, life-threatening medical emergency. In heatstroke, the body's temperature-regulating mechanisms are severely disabled. The body can no longer support its normal (98.6°F) temperature, and temperatures can soar to 105°F and beyond. Temperatures sustained at these heights begin to affect major organ systems of the body and result in the possibility of irreversible damage. Renal (kidney) and cardiac (heart) failure are not uncommon. At temperatures of 108°F and higher, irreversible brain damage can result. Profound shock and circulatory collapse are also symptomatic. The Keynote symptoms of heatstroke are:

1. Symptoms may occur suddenly, or develop gradually, but are preceded by general body weakness, dizziness/lightheadedness, headache, and nausea.
2. Before the absolute onset of fully developed symptoms, the victim may experience either a decrease in perspiration or its total cessation. This is a critical symptom!
3. The victim's skin is red, hot, and *dry* (the exact opposite of heat exhaustion).
4. The pulse rate bounds to 160 bpm or higher.
5. There is rapid respiration (20–30 inhalations per minute).
6. The victim is anxious, or listless, or unconscious.
7. The pupils of the eyes may at first contract (grow smaller) but will later dilate (become wider).

For emergency treatment, the victim/athlete must be stripped naked. Heatstroke is so profound a medical emergency, there is *no time for modesty*. The victim's body must be sponged (or immersed if possible) in cool water. Ice or cold packs may be applied. If the victim is immersed, *do not* add ice to the water. The victim should be massaged. Massage dilates the peripheral blood vessels in the skin, which assists heat regulation. In heatstroke, *never* administer any form of stimulant: alcohol, ammonia inhalants, etc. Also, always call for advanced medical assistance at the earliest moment.

The heatstroke victim's temperature should be monitored rectally, if possible. The body temperature must not be allowed to drop below 101°F as heatstroke's opposite, *hypothermia* (low body temperature), may result. Additionally, the victim must be treated for shock by elevating the legs and lowering the head to assist blood-to-brain circulation.

Homeopathic medicine provides several exceedingly effective remedies, which act to combat the symptoms of heatstroke and prevent an increase in the severity of symptoms. Of the remedies listed below, Belladonna and Glonoine are most frequently used, based upon the totality of symptoms presented.

It is not an uncommon complaint among athletes who have experienced heatstroke and recovered, to complain of nagging symptoms that recur in hot weather. Homeopathy can provide considerable aid and comfort for these individuals during the year's warm months, and help them back into the competitive or recreational activity. To illustrate: At age eleven, Paul S. had suffered heatstroke during a summer camping activity in late July. He had been initially treated at camp, then rushed to a local medical center for advanced care. Apparently recovered, he nevertheless was unable to resume a full schedule of normal activity during the summer months.

When Paul entered junior high, his natural athletic inclinations reasserted themselves and he chose to participate in winter basketball and spring track. To condition himself for these competitive activities, he ran three to five miles a day, year round. He found, however, that whenever the weather turned warm, he was "off-center" and often became sick with throbbing headaches and a general overall weakness.

The throbbing headaches he experienced so often indicated a need for Nat. mur., but his totality of symptoms also indicated Nat. carb. Both remedies, in 30x potencies, were given in alternate doses an hour apart for several days. Within a week, the usual pains and discomforts had subsided. By the end of the first summer, taking Nat. mur. and Nat. carb. in decreasing frequencies of alternating doses, the boy's condition returned to normal.

HOMEOPATHIC TREATMENT
Belladonna
Glonoine
Aconite
Gelsemium
Natrum Muriaticum (Nat. Mur.)
Natrum Carbonicum (Nat. Carb.)

Belladonna has the following Keynote symptoms:

1. The face is flushed bright red or bluish-red.
2. The skin is hot and glossy/shiny.
3. The victim is conscious and dizzy.
4. The victim complains of pain and throbbing, especially in the forehead.
5. The victim's breathing is heavy and labored.

Potency and Dosage: At the immediate onset of agreeing symptoms, give 5 1-grain tablets of Belladonna in the 200x or 200c potency. If not available, give the 30x, 15c, or 30c potency, every 15 minutes until symptoms subside, or advanced medical help arrives.

Glonoine is the homeopathic trituration of nitroglycerine. Its Keynote symptoms are:

1. The victim experiences mental confusion with dizziness.
2. The victim complains of a "heavy" head, with violent, throbbing, and bursting pains.

Potency and Dosage: At the immediate onset of agreeing symptoms, give 5 1-grain tablets of Glonoine in the 200x or 200c potency. If not available, give the 30x, 15c, or 30c potency, every 15 minutes until symptoms subside, or advanced medical help arrives.

Aconite has the following Keynote symptoms:

1. The victim experiences a feeling of fullness in the head.
2. The skin is hot.
3. The victim complains of bursting head pains with outward pressure made worse from sitting upright.
4. The victim is greatly anxious and may speak of the fear of death.

Potency and Dosage: 5 1-grain tablets in the high, 200c or 200x, potency. If unavailable, give 30x, 15c, or 30c potency every 15 minutes until outward symptoms subside, or until advanced medical support arrives.

Gelsemium has the following Keynote symptoms:

1. The face is hot and flushed red.
2. The victim is giddy as if drunk, on any attempt to move.
3. The victim complains of a band-like feeling around the head.
4. Head pain is located at the occipital (rear) of the skull.

Potency and Dosage: 5 1-grain tablets in the high, 200c or 200x, potency. If unavailable, give 30x, 15c, or 30c potency every 15 minutes until outward symptoms subside, or until advanced medical support arrives.

Nat. Mur. (the homeopathic trituration of sodium chloride) is one of the two most outstanding medicines for treating the debilitating aftereffects of heatstroke. Its application, of course, depends upon the totality of one Keynote symptom: The victim experiences a throbbing, blinding headache; "aches as if a thousand tiny hammers were pounding on the brain."

Potency and Dosage: Give 3 doses of Nat. mur. daily in the 6x–30x or 3c–15c potency for 2 or 3 days and await results. This treatment may be continued for two to four weeks if necessary.

Nat. Carb. (the homeopathic trituration of sodium carbonate) is yet another of the remedies often used in effectively dealing with the persistent, chronic aftereffects that heatstroke victims sometimes experience. Its Keynote symptoms are:

1. The victim experiences great debility caused by warm weather and summer heat.
2. A headache is made worse from exposure to the sun and the return of hot weather.

Potency and Dosage: Give 3 doses of Nat. carb. daily in the 6x–30x or 3c–15c potency for 2 or 3 days and await results. This treatment may be continued for two to four weeks if necessary.

Heat Exhaustion

During heat exhaustion, the blood pools in the capillaries of the skin while the body's heat-regulating mechanism attempts to expel its excess heat. The heart, lungs, and brain become oxygen deprived, while the lesser veins constrict as they compensate for the reduced volume of blood in circulation.

Heat exhaustion is actually the result of a gradual dehydration. Unlike heatstroke, which, though it offers early signals, can come suddenly, heat exhaustion may develop over several hours or several days. Blood volume, as it continues to be reduced, leads to a general and progressive weakness. The Keynote symptoms are:

1. The victim's skin is cool and moist, pale or white.
2. The victim's body temperature is usually normal (98.6°F) or only slightly elevated.
3. The victim may complain of general weakness, dizziness, or nausea, and sometimes of cramps in the muscles.
4. In advanced cases, the victim may faint, but will regain consciousness quickly after the legs are elevated above heart level.

Heat exhaustion, unlike its cousin, heatstroke, is generally not a medical emergency.

The athlete should be moved to a cool and sun-shaded location as soon as possible and his or her clothing loosened. It is unnecessary to strip the victim of heat exhaustion. Elevation of the victim's feet permits blood to circulate more freely to the brain. Fruit juices, or water with 1/4 to 1/2 teaspoon of dissolved table salt, given to the victim in small sips (never gulped) is of considerable benefit. Juice or water should not be given cold. The body may be cooled if the temperature is elevated, by applying cool, damp cloths, or by stimulating air circulation around the victim by fanning.

HOMEOPATHIC TREATMENT
Veratrum Album

Most heat exhaustion victims are greatly benefitted in a rapid recovery to normal function through **Veratrum Album**. The Keynote symptoms of this homeopathic medicine correspond to the general symptoms of heat exhaustion: cool, moist skin, coloration pale or white to bluish-white, nausea accompanied by vomiting, and cramping in the extremities.

Potency and Dosage: One dose of Veratrum album in 30x, 15c, or 30c potency (lesser potencies are also beneficial if midrange potencies are un-available) every 15 minutes until symptoms subside.

Heat Cramps

Heat cramp comes as a result of the profuse sweating in which sodium (salt) is lost during sports activities performed in temperatures exceeding 100°F. This occurs especially among athletes who have not properly conditioned themselves in training to work through such temperatures.

The prevention of heat cramp is more effective than its treatment. All people who participate in sports activities should precondition themselves for warm weather and high humidity conditions. Dress should be appropriate and noninsulating, permitting perspiration and body heat to escape easily from the skin's surface. An adequate intake of fluids is essential; the best fluid is plain, pure water.

There is a great deal of misunderstanding among athletes on the proper use of salt as a preventive against heat-stress illnesses. Very few athletes lose any appreciable quantity of sodium (salt) in perspiration. Athletes *do not require* supplemental salt. Salt is a Catch 22 situation: Too much salt retains water in the body—an undesirable condition. Too little salt is also dangerous. The body maintains an optimum sodium balance. Going on a "salt-free" diet (defined by the medical profession as the intake of 5 mg. sodium or less per food item), as some amateur and professional athletes may do mistakenly, can destroy the body's sodium balance. Its reaction can then be dehydration and loss of potassium. As the general diet of athletes contains sufficient quantities of sodium, there is seldom a good reason for any athlete to add additional salt in the form of salt tablets, or by shaking extra salt on food.

Salt tablets, unless they are enteric coated, dissolve in the stomach rather than the small intestine and often cause stomach erosion or distress.

In recent years, several commercial food companies have introduced into the athletic market drinks that contain the mineral salts and sugar normally lost during warm or hot weather exertion. These products are meant to maintain the normal and essential balance of electrolytes in the body.

Today, the majority of sports medicine specialists, coaches, trainers, and nutritionists recommend that, if these products are used at all, they be diluted at least 50/50 if not even 3 to 1 with water. The Keynote symptoms of heat cramp are:

1. The onset is sudden.

2. The victim may lie flat with legs flexed (due to abdominal cramping) or roll from the extreme pain of muscular spasms.

3. Arms and legs (extremities) are most commonly affected, but abdominal muscles may be subject to spasm.

4. Body temperature remains normal (98.6°F) but the skin is pale and moist.

Left untreated, heat cramps may continue for hours, greatly debilitating the athlete. General treatment in heat cramp is the same as in heat exhaustion. Firm massage over the affected muscle, or firm pressure may assist in relieving the spasms.

HOMEOPATHIC TREATMENT
Magnesia Phosphorica (Mag. Phos.)

A well-known homeopathic antispasmodic (anticramping) remedy, **Mag. Phos.** is a trituration of the mineral salt, magnesium phosphate. Mag. phos. has been proved in innumerable situations to relieve muscle spasms within a few minutes following administration.

Potency and Dosage: Give 15 to 20 1-grain tablets dissolved in water (hot water seems to boost the rapidity of Mag. phos's anticramping action) every 15 minutes in half-glass doses.

---

16. Guidelines for long distance runners appear in *British Medical Journal*, 5 May 1984, 288:1356-8.

CHAPTER NINE

GASTROINTESTINAL TRAUMAS

Topics Covered

Diarrhea
Food Poisoning
Nausea and Vomiting

Diarrhea

One of the most valuable reference textbooks on homeopathic prescribing, *Boericke's Materia Medica with Repertory,* lists some one hundred and fourteen medications for diarrhea, each based upon the totality of symptoms presented in the individual. In this section, only those remedies most often called upon will be considered.

Diarrhea is indeed an unpleasant complaint, especially for athletes when it occurs in association with competition. However, at times diarrhea is one of the methods the body employs to rapidly rid itself of toxic material, bacteria, and other irritants.

An occasional loose stool, or even two loose bowel movements a day is certainly no cause for alarm and may, in fact, be natural. The looseness and frequency of the stool is dependent upon several factors, and diet certainly is one. Today, probably due to many articles written on health and nutrition for athletes and the general sporting public, more and more of us are adding crude fiber, bran, fruits and vegetables, and even unbuttered, unsalted popcorn to our daily diets. Popcorn, by the way, is an excellent addition to the diet, especially without additional salt (the Western diet has too much salt) or butter (a source of undesirable cholesterol and saturated fatty acids). Popcorn, bran, and other fibers absorb large quantities of water in the bowel, swell, and move wastes more rapidly through the intestinal tract.

The important consideration in diarrhea is frequency of bowel movement. Several very loose, highly fluid, sometimes fetid stools a day is a symptom of acute diarrhea. Athletes prior to competition occasionally experience a "nervous diarrhea"– an annoying and troubling condition.

In the homeopathic approach to diarrhea, the prescriber must study each listed remedy closely and select that remedy which most closely matches the symptoms. Following these Keynote symptoms, the prescriber will almost certainly be able to correct the problem quickly.

HOMEOPATHIC TREATMENT
Arsenicum Album (Arsenicum Alb.)
Veratum Album (Veratum Alb.)
China
Podophyllum
Colocynthis
Croton Tiglium
Dulcamara
Nitric Acid

The first two homeopathic remedies, Arsenicum alb. and Veratum alb., cover the majority of the most common symptoms of acute diarrhea.

The Keynote symptoms for **Arsenicum Alb.** are:

1. Stools are small in quantity.
2. The victim is restless, anguished, and intolerant of pain.
3. Considerable thirst accompanies the diarrhea, but only for small amounts of liquids, with a frequent desire to drink.
4. This diarrhea is associated with great weakness and prostration.

Potency and Dosage: Any potency is effective from the lower 6x and 3c, to the midrange potencies of 30x and 30c. Lower potencies may be repeated, 1 dose every 15 to 30 minutes in the initial severe, acute stage, dosage reduced to 1 dose every 2 to 3 hours until symptoms subside. The higher, midrange potencies may be given once every 30 minutes for the first hour, then once every 2 to 3 hours until symptoms abate.

Veratum Alb. has the following Keynote symptoms:

1. Stools are extremely loose and large in quantity (in contrast with the small quantity for Arsenicum alb.).
2. There is *no* restlessness, anguish, or intolerance to pain.
3. The victim is very thirsty for large quantities of cold water.
4. Great prostration follows each passing stool.

Veratum alb. also has diarrhea accompanied by vomiting which is profuse and violent. Stools are also expelled with great force.

Potency and Dosage: Follow the same prescribing information as for Arsenicum alb.

The next five homeopathic remedies aid specific symptoms. The potency and dosage are the same as for Arsenicum alb.

For *China,* the Keynote symptom is frequent watery stools with gripping abdominal pains.

Podophyllum has the following Keynote symptoms:

1. There is morning diarrhea *without pain.*
2. The stool is greenish, watery, with a strong, decayed odor.
3. The stool is expelled with great force – gushing.

Colocynthis has the following Keynote symptoms:

1. There are cutting, agonizing pains in the abdomen causing the victim to bend over double to relieve the pain.

2. Pain is relieved by pressing directly and firmly on the abdomen.
3. Stools are jelly-like and brown, or yellowish.

Croton Tig. has the following Keynote symptoms:

1. Diarrhea occurs more commonly in the warm summer months.
2. Stools are large and watery.
3. There is great urging to the stool, which is always forcefully expelled.
4. Gurgling may be heard in the intestines.
5. Drinking liquids increases the diarrhea.

For *Dulcamara* there are the following Keynote symptoms:

1. The stool is green, watery, slimy, often bloody and spotted with clumps of white mucus.
2. There is diarrhea especially during the summer, occurring especially whenever the warm weather turns suddenly chilled.

Some athletes who have taken, or are currently taking, a course of anti-biotic therapy for a bacterial infection may experience altered intestinal transit. Antibiotics may increase the normal intestinal transit time of fecal material by modifying the normal stool bacteria resulting in stimulation of the smooth muscle wall of the intestine. *Nitric Acid* in homeopathic dilution is *the* remedy of choice in antibiotic-caused diarrhea and will promptly relieve the condition.

Potency and Dosage: Give 1 dose (5 1-grain tablets, or 6 to 8 pellets) of the 30x, 15c, or 30c potency every 2 to 3 hours for a maximum dosage of 9 repetitions. The condition should be relieved within a matter of only a few hours.

Food Poisoning

In the sudden onset of diarrhea, nausea, cramping, or violent abdominal pains, food poisoning should be suspected. This is especially true if several members of an athletic team develop similar symptom patterns.

Most forms of food poisoning are the result of improperly refrigerated protein foods, dairy products, beef, pork, poultry, and eggs. Foods may also be contaminated through improper storage or handling.

Staphylococcal enterotoxin produces *ptomaine poisoning*. Its symptoms develop within one to eight hours of eating contaminated food and generally abate within 8 hours without treatment. Fortunately, most food poisonings are self-limiting.

ADVISORY WARNING: Should severe gastrointestinal symptoms – nausea, vomiting, diarrhea – be accompanied by progressive muscle weakness, blurring vision, and difficulty in swallowing or speaking, botulism must be suspected. This is an ACUTE MEDICAL EMERGENCY.

HOMEOPATHIC TREATMENT
Arsenicum Album (Arsenicum Alb.)
Pyrogen

The Keynote symptoms for **Arsenicum Alb.** are:

1. There is burning pain in the gastrointestinal tract. (This is the most common symptom in determining Arsenicum alb.)
2. The abdomen is painful, swollen, and distended.
3. There are nausea and retching and, after eating or drinking, vomiting.
4. The sight or smell of food is offensive to the victim.
5. Stools are dark, extremely odorous, and small in quantity.
6. On the least exertion the victim experiences great weakness and debility.

Potency and Dosage: 1 dose every 30 minutes for the first hour, and continued every 2 to 3 hours, as required until symptoms subside. Give Arsenicum alb. in 6x–30x or 30c potencies.

Pyrogen has the following Keynote symptoms:

1. There are intolerable cramping and cutting pains in the abdomen.

2. The diarrhea is painless and involuntary.

3. Stools are large and black with a distinctive decaying odor.

4. Vomiting occurs after drinking water; the vomitus resembles coffee grounds.

Potency and Dosage: Administer Pyrogen as for Arsenicum alb. above.

Nausea and Vomiting

ADVISORY WARNING: Any persistent nausea and vomiting in athletes under the age of 18, especially, but not limited to, occurring after a viral infection such as a cold, influenza, or chicken pox, may be suggestive of *Reye's syndrome*. Reye's (pronounced ryes) is a disease of unknown cause that most commonly affects children and adolescents. It most often occurs in the late autumn and winter, from November to March. Besides nausea and vomiting, personality changes frequently occur: forgetfulness, lethargy, agitation or combativeness, disorientation. REYE'S SYNDROME IS A LIFE-THREATENING MEDICAL EMERGENCY. Do not administer any medication. Contact a physician or hospital emergency room immediately.

HOMEOPATHIC TREATMENT
Ipecac
Tobacum
Cocculus

Most people think of **Ipecac** as a thick syrup given to small children who have ingested poison. In fact, many pharmacies make syrup of ipecac available at cost or free of charge to parents with small children as an emergency treatment for poisoning accidents.

Since ipecac (ipecacuanha) produces vomiting, its homeopathic trituration *reverses* this process. Its Keynote symptoms are:

1. There is continuous, persistent nausea accompanied by copious salivation.

2. There is persistent and continuous vomiting.
3. Vomiting does not relieve nausea. This is ipecac's most important symptom.

Potency and Dosage: Ipecac works best in its lower potencies. The 3x and 6x (3c) potencies are the most effective. Give 1 dose every 15 to 30 minutes in acute nausea and vomiting, reducing the frequency of dosages as symptoms subside.

Tobacum is a useful homeopathic remedy made from raw tobacco leaves. It is an effective cure of nausea and vomiting, and a remedy frequently used in treating motion sickness which some athletes may experience, whenever its Keynote symptoms agree:

1. There is wave upon wave of dizziness, made worse from any and all movement.
2. There is a feeling of faintness accompanied by a sick and sinking sensation in the pit of the stomach.
3. There is great dizziness.

Potency and Dosage: Tobacum is effective in all low and midrange potencies (6x–30x or 30c). Give 1 dose every 30 minutes in acute cases, reducing dosage as symptoms subside.

Cocculus (also highly effective in alleviating motion sickness) has the following Keynote symptoms:

1. All symptoms are increased by motion.
2. The head feels heavy and empty.
3. There is dizziness and nausea, especially when riding in a moving vehicle or on sitting upright.
4. There is nausea from motion, or from viewing moving objects.
5. There is a total distaste for food or drinks.
6. There is a metallic taste in the mouth.

Potency and Dosage: The same as for Tobacum.

CHAPTER TEN

SKIN TROUBLES

Topics Covered

Boils
Carbuncles
Eczema
Sunburn
Fungus Infections: Ringworm
"Wrestlers' Warts"

Boils

Boils tend to be a rather common sports-related skin condition, especially among young wrestlers.

A boil, also known as a *furuncle,* is an acutely tender, inflamed nodule occurring anywhere on the skin and caused by staphylococcal bacteria. The most common skin sites where boils occur are the face, neck, chest, and buttocks.

HOMEOPATHIC TREATMENT
Hypericum Tincture and Internal Potency
Tarentula Cubensis

Having treated boils homeopathically without a single failure for over twelve years, I have found the most direct and simple treatment appears to be the use of **Hypericum,** in either its tincture or in its internal potency. It can also be used in a combination of both forms. One often needs to do little more than paint the surface of the boil with undiluted Hypericum tincture and cover it with a sterile gauze pad and surgical or adhesive tape. Reapplication of the tincture twice to three times a day is normally all the treatment required. There is no need to apply moist, hot cloths to hasten suppuration (drainage), to have it lanced, or to use antibiotic ointments or antibiotics internally.

Admittedly anecdotal, the following two case histories will clearly demonstrate the rapidity and efficacy of homeopathic treatment of boils in young athletes.

A junior high school wrestler, age 13, was brought to me by his father with a boil on his right shoulder about 8 mm. in diameter. When I first saw him, the boil was very near suppuration stage. Otherwise in excellent health, the boy had no previous history of boils. Treatment consisted of applying Hypericum tincture liberally, undiluted, directly onto the boil and for several millimeters of surrounding healthy skin. The boil was then covered with sterile gauze and taped. The boy's father was given a 1/4-oz. bottle of Hypericum tincture with instructions to reapply it twice daily and telephone with the results. The father called at the end of the second day to report that the boil had just suppurated and begun to drain. Upon a brief follow-up visit on the third day, the boy's shoulder showed only smooth, healthy tissue with just a hint of redness.

A 16-year-old high school wrestler indicated that he had had numbers of boils, occurring on various parts of his body, over the past two years. An ardent wrestler, no doubt he was picking up staphylococcal bacteria from the wrestling mat, and the boils developed when bacteria entered the skin through minute cuts or abrasions. Normally, the skin is an impermeable membrane through which bacteria cannot pass. Once damaged, however, bacteria, which are always present on the skin's surface, enter and produce infection. In this case, the boil was newly formed, about 30 mm. across (the size of a small hen's egg) and located on the posterior thigh midway between the buttocks and knee. Again, treatment consisted of a liberal application of undiluted Hypericum tincture and a gauze dressing well moistened with additional Hypericum tincture. As the boil was nowhere nearing the suppuration stage, Hypericum 30x was given by mouth, 3 1-grain tablets to be dissolved under the tongue every 4 hours for 2 days. On the second day following initial treatment, the teenager returned for evaluation. The boil had shrunk from 30 mm. to 10 mm. without suppuration, although a central core of pus was clearly visible. With the wooden stick of a cotton applicator rolled gently from both edges of the boil, the core was expelled. Additional Hypericum tincture was applied and the wound redressed. A brief revisit on the third day showed no sign of the former infection. Hypericum internally, in potency, was discontinued; no further treatment was required.

Hypericum tincture normally brings boils to rapid resolution. Its powerful anti-infection action often ripens the boil, promotes suppuration and drainage, and rapid healing without pain or effort.

Potency and Dosage: Apply the undiluted tincture locally, 2 to 4 times daily as required. Soaking a sterile gauze pad with additional Hypericum is considered standard practice. As an adjunct therapy, Hypericum may be given internally in the lower (6x, 3c or 6c) to the midrange 30x, 15c or 30c potencies, to be discontinued as symptoms lessen.

I often hesitate to inform patients of the composition of **Tarentula Cubensis,** which so often does yeoman's work in boils. It is prepared homeopathically from the venom of the Cuban spider (tarantula). Undiluted, in its nonhomeopathic trituration, Tarentula cubensis produces local abscesses of a distinctive purple coloration accompanied by stinging and burning pains. These symptoms are accompanied by localized redness and swelling. Taken together, this symptom grouping is the "classic" symptom of a boil. As proven in decades of clinical experience, that which causes a condition to appear in the healthy body can, in its homeopathic microdilution, cure that condition.

To illustrate: One evening, a Doctor of Dental Surgery with whom I was acquainted called to ask if I would see his son. The boy was a handsome, athletic 15-year-old, a gymnast and swimmer. Having never met me, the boy was somewhat shy, and more especially so considering the location of the boil. He had developed a 10 mm. marble-sized boil in his groin, immediately adjacent to his testicle. The infection was extremely tender, painful to the touch, and made movement extremely uncomfortable.

Hypericum, in undiluted tincture form, would have been appropriate here, as it is in most cases of boils. However, the location of the boil—near the tender scrotum—and its physical appearance—a distinctive purplish color—best indicated another remedy. Tarentula cubensis in 30x potency was administered, 5 1-grain tablets dissolved under the tongue to be repeated every 4 hours until local symptoms abated. I did not see the boy again. However, his father called about a week later to relate that the boil had "simply disappeared" within three days following Tarentula. Of course, no further treatment was required.

Potency and Dosage: The 30x or 30c–200c potency may be given. The 30x or 30c potencies may be given 3 to 4 times daily, as required. The high 200c potency should be repeated no more than twice.

Carbuncle

Perhaps the first cousin to the boil is the carbuncle. A carbuncle, which occurs most commonly on the neck, is a boil cluster, as large as 50 mm. (2 inches) or more with multiple pus-filled cores. Carbuncles produce deep-tissue suppuration and are often slow to heal.

Predisposing factors may underlie the formation of carbuncles—diabetes mellitus and other diseases. Therefore, the root cause for this predisposition should be considered in consultation with a health care practitioner. Normal treatment of carbuncles consists of oral antibiotics such as penicillinase-resistant penicillin or erythromycin for up to three or four months. As with the boil, the normal infective agent is staphylococcus.

It is not recommended that the nonphysician treat a carbuncle due to the depth and extent of the infection and the possibility of serious underlying causative factors (such as diabetes). Homeopathic treatment for carbuncles is highly effective. However, this should be accomplished only by the trained health care practitioner.

HOMEOPATHIC TREATMENT
Hepar Sulphuris (Hepar. Sulph.)

If Hypericum is unavailable, or the boil should not show the distinctive purple hue denoting Tarentula cubensis, **Hepar. Sulph.** may be well employed in its lower potencies (which act to promote suppuration and drainage).

Potency and Dosage: 6x or 3c, repeated every 2 to 3 hours as required to produce suppuration.

Hepar sulph. is most effective when used before pus has obviously formed. It has the power, in unformed, unripe boils, to absorb the infection completely, especially if the boil is exquisitely tender and painful to any pressure.

> ADVISORY WARNING: Do not use Hepar sulph. if the patient is experiencing *otitis media* (inflammation of the middle ear). Hepar sulph. in low potencies so rapidly hastens suppuration that damage to the eardrum may result.

Eczema

The homeopathic medical profession recognizes two types of eczema, *constitutional* and *acquired*. Of the two types, only acquired eczema will be presented here. Constitutional eczema, or so called chronic eczema, is considered by homeopaths to be a condition of delayed allergy because it is most frequently seen in infancy and continues on well into adulthood. Constitutional eczema is also referred to as *atopic dermatitis*.

Treatment of three conditions will be discussed: eczema of the scalp, flaking skin eruptions, and wet ("weeping") eruptions.

HOMEOPATHIC TREATMENT
Calcium Carbonate (Calc. Carb.)
Natrum Muriaticum (Nat. Mur.)
Sulphur
Arsenicum Iodatum
Natrum Sulphuricum (Nat. Sulph.)
Petroleum
Graphites

A common skin disorder in both infants and adults, scalp eczema is characterized by chalk-white to yellowish crusts on the scalp. This form of eczema generally rapidly yields to homeopathic *Calc. Carb.* (Calcium carbonate) in 30x, 15c, or 30c potencies taken in once-weekly doses of 5 1-grain tablets. Calc. carb. should not be repeated too frequently; therefore once-weekly doses are preferred.

The Keynote symptoms of Calc. carb. help guide its selection as the most appropriate remedy:

1. The scalp condition increases in severity during cold, wet weather.
2. The scalp condition is better for dry warmth.

A similar skin condition to that described above occurs in adults at the hair line rather than on the head itself. Here, *Nat. Mur.* (the homeopathic trituration of sodium chloride) will almost always clear up the condition. Nat. mur. is also exceptionally effective in eliminating any skin condition occurring on the hair-covered parts of the body when the eruptions are oily or greasy, or in crusting, dry eruptions that occur in the bends or flexor surfaces of the joints and behind the ears.

The Keynote symptoms of Nat. mur. are:

1. The skin condition is worse from heat or warmth.
2. The condition is better from cool weather.

Potency and Dosage: Midrange to high potencies appear to work most effectively in Nat. mur. Give a 5-tablet, 1-grain dose of 30x, 15c, or 30c once daily for a week and await results. The high 200c potency has shown considerable effectiveness and may be given in a 5-tablet, 1-grain dose once weekly for several weeks. Stop treatment as symptoms subside, regardless of the potency selected.

At times, even the best selected remedy requires a "boost" to assist in its curative action. Should the best chosen Keynote remedy fail to provide complete relief, consider *Sulphur* in 30x, 15c, or 30c potency, taken as directed above. Sulphur in its crude form produces flaking, dry, and scaly skin eruptions that itch and are made worse from bathing and scratching. Therefore, in its triturated homeopathic potencies, sulphur often reverses the condition.

Arsenicum Iodatum should not be confused with Arsenicum album. The actions of these two medicines are not the same.

The Keynote symptoms or Arsenicum iodatum in skin eruptions are:

1. There is itching, which accompanies the eruption.
2. The eruption is scaly, dry, and rough.
3. Flakes are small and, when they loosen, the skin beneath is raw in appearance, and watery.

Potency and Dosage: Arsenicum iodatum should not be used below the 3c or 6x potency. The midrange, 30x potency appears to have a significant healing effect. Give 1 3-tablet dose 2 to 3 times a day for a maximum of 9 doses and await results

Nat. Sulph., the homeopathic preparation of sodium sulphate, is considered a tissue or cell salt. Nat. sulph. is differentiated from Arsenicum iodatum by the appearance of the skin eruption in the following Keynote symptoms:

1. There are medium- to large-size flakes on the skin surface (in Arsenicum iodatum the flakes are small).
2. The flakes are normally yellowish in color.
3. As the plaques (flakes) slough away, the skin beneath is red, shiny and dry (compare Arsenicum iodatum's watery skin surface).

Potency and Dosage: Nat. sulph. may be used in its low, 6x or 3c potency, with doses repeated frequently (there are no adverse effects), or in its midrange, 30x or 15c potency, less frequently, as needed.

Petroleum is prepared from crude oil. In its homeopathic potencies, Petroleum frequently relieves eruptions that are dry and scaly, or at times moist when they occur during the colder winter months. The skin condition which Petroleum best addresses disappears during the warm weather of summer and early fall.

Potency and Dosage: 6x or 3c to be repeated as needed until the condition begins to clear, in 3 to 4 doses daily. Petroleum has demonstrated exceptional healing value in the midrange 30x or 15c potency taken 2 to 3 times daily for 3 to 4 days and stopped as symptoms subside.

Like Petroleum, *Graphites* is a carbon-based remedy which homeopathic medicine has found exceptionally useful in all skin conditions where the following Keynote symptoms occur:

1. The skin breaks open and "weeps" a thick, honeylike discharge.
2. The discharge dries to form a thick, yellow to light-brown crust.

Graphites eruptions are most likely to occur on the palms of the hands, between fingers and toes, or around the genitals and mouth. At times the eruptions will occur around the nipples.

The Keynote symptoms of Graphites are often significant in leading to its selection as the most appropriate remedy:

1. The eruption is worse from warmth.
2. In women, the eruption is worse during and immediately following menstruation (apparently from the hormonal changes occurring at this time).
3. The eruption is better from the application of cold.

To illustrate its use: A retired Air Force major and ardent golfer developed a localized eruption on the fleshy portion of the thumbs of both hands. The condition was unsightly and irritating and, he indicated, adversely affected his game. The eruption at first appeared as a pinhead distribution of blisters that itched intensely then broke open to ooze a thick, yellowish discharge. He had applied a topical 0.5% hydrocortisone ointment without results and had been given a prescription cortisone ointment by a fellow golfer, again without results. The Keynote symptoms of Graphites were all present: worse from warmth (golf is played in the heat of the summer months), and the eruption broke open and oozed a thick, honeylike discharge. Graphites in 3x potency was given in 5 1-grain tablets, 4 times daily. Within one week the most prominent symptoms had subsided, and within two weeks, all signs of the eruption had vanished. The following summer, he again experienced a similar condition, and, again, Graphites 3x produced a clear skin within one week.

Potency and Dosage: Use the lower potencies, 3x, 6x, or 3c. Graphites may also be used externally as an ointment with significant results when applied several times daily. The disadvantage of this approach is that Graphites ointment is black and stains clothing.

Sunburn

The ever-increasing interest in outdoor activities places more and more people in danger of frank overexposure to the ultraviolet rays of the sun. This is even truer today than just ten years ago, since some scientific research has suggested that various common chemicals in use worldwide have reduced and continue to reduce the ozone layer of the atmosphere. This reduction in the earth's balance permits the damaging ultraviolet rays to penetrate the atmosphere more easily. Those outdoor enthusiasts who do not take the proper preventive precautions can well expect skin damage.

Reaction to the sun varies. Dark-skinned and black athletes have more melanin, a protective pigment, in the skin and are therefore less susceptible to sunburn and skin damage than those who are light-complexioned. But even dark skin, or a deep, golden tan do not guarantee total protection from the sun.

Sunlight, and hence the concentration of ultraviolet rays, is most intense between midmorning and early afternoon and in the summer. Cloudy, overcast days do not offer protection either. The sun's ultraviolet rays penetrate the overhead cloud layer and bounce off objects on the ground. Boaters, swimmers, fishermen, and water skiers are frequently victims of severe sunburn because water reflects 85% of the sun's rays directly back onto the skin. The same fact is true of snow, and it is not uncommon for snow skiers to become burned on the unprotected portions of the face.

The best "treatment" for sunburn is prevention—not to become burned at all. Currently, the best protection is offered by products called sunscreens whose major ingredient is PABA—a B vitamin, para-aminobenzoic acid—matched to the degree of fairness and sensitivity of the skin. These PABA products vary from SPF (Sun Protection Factor) of 4 (lowest) to 24 (highest). An odd fact, however, is that in some unusually sensitive persons, PABA may actually promote burning. Severe sunburn and continued overexposure to the sun will, over a period of years, cause premature skin aging, severe and irreversible wrinkling and sagging that even plastic surgery cannot repair, and there is the ever-present danger of developing actinic keratoses — small, scaly patches on overexposed skin that may predispose one to skin cancers.

If a first- or second-degree sunburn occurs and one is caught without the proper homeopathic remedy, vitamin E or aloe vera gel are both very useful products. Vitamin E is quite probably the best nonhomeopathic remedy in burns. Applied to the surface of the skin, vitamin E quickly removes pain and rapidly heals the damaged tissue. Aloe vera, a succulent plant whose juice contains a strong antiburn property, is also of considerable value in treating minor burns. One or the other should be applied liberally several times a day, to promote rapid healing. Vitamin E is *preferred* in more severe first- and second-degree burns.

Here are a couple of case histories in which homeopathic treatment of sunburn yielded rapid, satisfying results:

As the medical officer at a summer camp, I was called upon to treat one of the most severe cases of second-degree sunburn I have ever seen. The boy was 14. He entered the relative cool of the Health Lodge, walking stiffly and obviously in great pain. He carried his white T-shirt in his hand. The boy was just the type to sunburn easily — with blonde, almost white hair and penetrating blue eyes. All across his chest, upper arms, and back was brilliant red skin with a large crop of clear, fluid-filled blisters ranging in diameter from pinheads to pencil erasers. He could scarcely move, and the pressure of clothing or touch was unbearable.

The boy was accompanied by a camp leader who had, as a first aid treatment, liberally applied a greasy, commercial burn ointment. Before anything could be done, this had to be removed — a procedure that proved excruciatingly painful for the boy. Once his skin was free of the ointment, I applied a solution of Urtica urens tincture, diluted to a 10% strength with water, and dabbed it liberally onto the damaged skin. Within five minutes of the first application, the boy calmed down considerably. A second application was made, and Urtica urens 30x given by mouth. A few minutes later, the boy was completely calm — his pain relieved.

I gave the leader a small bottle of diluted tincture and instructions to apply it every hour and to see me immediately if the blisters opened. The next afternoon, barely 24 hours later, the boy returned. He was now wearing his T-shirt, whereas the day before he couldn't tolerate even the slightest pressure on his skin. The blisters, which had varied from pinhead size to the diameter of my little fingernail, were nearly gone. And, two days later on a return visit, the skin showed only the slightest rosy tinge, without a single blister. Urtica urens in homeopathic potency externally and internally had done its job well. Cantharis, internally, had I had any, might well have done an even better clearing.

The second case of sunburn occurred late in the summer of 1984. A 15-year-old water skier came to me with severe second-degree sunburn on his lips.

Anyone engaged in outdoor activities, regardless of the time of year, and especially water skiers, fishermen, and snow skiers, should wear an SPF sunscreen lip balm. But, often, this simplest of preventive measures is the most overlooked.

The boy's lips were not only covered with water-filled vesicles and enormously swollen, but they burned also. Burning is a definite indication for the use of Cantharis, although blister formation without burning does not preclude its use. The boy was given Cantharis 30c in 5 1-grain doses to be taken every 3 hours of the waking day, for one day, reduced to 3 times daily, the second day. When the boy reappeared for a brief revisit on the third day, all signs of blistering had vanished.

HOMEOPATHIC TREATMENT
Calendula Lotion
Hypericum Lotion
Urtica Urens Lotion
Cantharis
Causticum

The first three homeopathically prepared products listed above, applied on the skin as lotions, work rapidly to relieve the pain of sunburn and assist in establishing rapid and natural healing.

Calendula Lotion contains 10% concentration of Calendula extract (from the African marigold) and is one of the finest products available for minor sunburn. *Hypericum Lotion,* made from the herb St. John's wort, is nearly specific to any skin injury affecting nerves, as in first-degree and minor second-degree burns. *Urtica Urens Lotion* is a homeopathic preparation of the dwarf stinging nettle, with a long history of success in treating minor first- and second-degree sunburn. Each lotion, varying in its concentration of plant extracts from 2% to 10%, is nongreasy and nonstaining.

In treating minor sunburn, two homeopathic remedies stand out, Cantharis and Causticum.

Cantharis is made from a trituration of the Spanish beetle. It acts rapidly to relieve the pain of any burn and is exceptionally useful in treating both the pain and the blistering produced by second-degree sunburn.

Potency and Dosage: 6x–30x or 30c potencies are best. 3 1-grain tablets placed under the tongue and dissolved every 15 to 30 minutes, as needed to relieve pain, or as pain returns.

Causticum is a homeopathic mineral remedy, slaked lime and bisulphate of potash. A powerful pain-relieving remedy, Causticum often rivals Cantharis in its ability to relieve burn pain. It does not, however, have the blister-eliminating power of Cantharis.

Potency and Dosage: 6x–30x or 30c potencies are best. 3 1-grain tablets placed under the tongue and dissolved every 15 to 30 minutes as needed to relieve pain, or as pain returns.

Fungus Infections: Ringworm

Ringworm is nothing more than a superficial fungal infection of the skin. Caused by fungi called *dermatophytes,* it invades only the first or so-called dead layer of the skin, and sometimes affects the nails and scalp. The clinical names for ringworm as it appears on various parts of the body are quite impressive: *tinea corporis* (ringworm of the body), *tinea pedis* (athlete's foot), *tinea unguium* (ringworm of the nails), *tinea capitis* (ringworm of the scalp), and finally *tinea cruris* (ringworm of the groin).

Generally ringworm is self-curative. Left untreated, it will go away on its own. Most athletes, however, are unwilling, understandably so, to permit one of these conditions to linger on for weeks or months. Because they are contagious the athlete is not allowed to compete in most athletic competitions until treatment has begun. The only real danger of any of the *tinea* infections is the possibility of developing a more serious secondary bacterial infection. And, of course, the term "worm" has nothing whatsoever to do with an actual parasite burrowing under the top layer of the skin. The term describes the appearance of the infection. Ringworm is a gradually extending lesion with a scaly, slightly raised red border that forms a ring shape. It extends outward and clears from the center outward. Thus its name.

As is true in all unhealthy conditions of the body, prevention is always preferable to cure. Athlete's foot is likely to occur when the feet become wet from perspiration following a heavy workout; from hot, humid weather activities; and from wearing improperly fitting shoes. Athletes should strive to keep their feet dry by exposing them to the open air whenever possible, and wearing socks that wick moisture away from the skin. *Tinea cruris,* that appears on the upper, inner portions of the thighs and in the groin, can also often be prevented by wearing loose-fitting clothing that breathes, and changing underwear or athletic support clothing whenever they become damp following workouts or competition.

HOMEOPATHIC TREATMENT
Sepia
Tellurium
Graphites
Sulphur
Rhus Toxicodendron (Rhus Tox.)

Homeotherapeutics provide effective treatments for ringworm, wherever it appears on the body. The Keynote symptoms listed under each remedy will guide the user in selecting the most appropriate remedy.

Ringworm generally is rapidly cured by **Sepia** in uncomplicated infections. The Keynote symptoms follow:

1. Patches are circular and scaly and brown to reddish brown in color.
2. The affected skin itches and burns after scratching.

Potency and Dosage: Employ midrange to high potencies infrequently. Preferred potencies are 30x, 15c, 30c, or 200c. In the 200c potency, 3 doses once daily for 3 days is generally sufficient. If necessary, Sepia 200c may be repeated following a 2- or 3-day interval for another 3 days. In the midrange potencies, give 1 3-tablet, 1-grain dose 2 to 3 times daily for a week.

Tellurium has the following Keynote symptoms:

1. The skin is scaly and dry with a definite circular marking.
2. The lesion is red more than brown, making the lesion's ring(s) stand out prominently.
3. Small patches of fluid-filled blisters may appear on the rings and break to ooze a thin liquid.

Potency and Dosage: Midrange to high potencies employed infrequently: 30x, 15c, 30c, or 200c. Repeat as indicated under Sepia.

Graphites has the following Keynote symptoms:

1. Thick scaly patches appear on the skin.
2. Patches break and ooze a thick, honeylike fluid.

Potency and Dosage: Graphites is best employed in its lower 3x potency. Give 3 1-grain tablets to be dissolved under the tongue every 2 or 3 hours as needed until a significant improvement occurs.

Sulphur is the remedy to consider if the best-selected remedies fail to provide rapid and significant relief, or if the following Keynote symptoms are present:

1. There is extreme itching.
2. There is excessive aggravation from warmth.

Potency and Dosage: Use midrange to high potencies, 30x, 15c, 30c, or 200c, as under Sepia.

Ringworm of the scalp often yields nicely to **Rhus Toxicodendron** when the irritation is moist or runny. Employ Rhus tox. 200c as indicated under Sepia. Rhus tox. follows Sepia well.

"Wrestlers' Warts"

A rather common condition that afflicts many young wrestlers is warts. These warts may appear anywhere on the body, but most commonly they appear on the face (flat warts) and elbows. Since warts are viral and contagious, many schools will not allow wrestlers who complain of them to compete.

As homeopathy individualizes diseases by the unique symptom pictures they present, rather than their causes, it is necessary to carefully differentiate between their appearance in order to determine the best treatment.

HOMEOPATHIC TREATMENT
Dulcamara
Natrum Sulphuricum
Antimonium Crudum
Nitric Acid
Causticum
Graphites

Flat, transparent warts are often nearly invisible in direct light but are more readily seen in reflected light, appearing far more frequently on the backs of the hands rather than other parts of the body. The remedy of choice is **Dulcamara**.

Potency and Dosage: In flat, transparent warts, Dulcamara is best administered in the 12x–30x or 6c–30c potencies, twice daily until symptoms subside. These warts may also require an additional homeopathic constitutional treatment. The inclusion of a 30x trituration of **Natrum Sulphuricum** (Nat. sulph.), together with the direct, symptomatic treatment using Dulcamara, will eliminate the peculiar predisposition to these types of warts.

Dark, translucent warts appear as fleshy protrusions on the skin, dark-colored and large. Their fleshy appearance creates the illusion that they are filled with fluid.

Potency and Dosage: In flat, dark, translucent warts, the homeopathic treatment of choice is again Dulcamara in the 6c or 12x potencies, given twice daily until symptoms subside. As with flat, transparent warts, Nat. sulph. can be beneficial as described above.

The most typical type of wart, the hard wart with its elevated and hard, corny appearance, was almost poetically described by Lewis Thomas, M.D., as springing up "like morning mushrooms" on otherwise healthy skin and having all the appearance of impregnable fortresses providing defense against the outside world.

A wart is nothing more than the complex reproductive apparatus of a virus. And, while allopathic medicine uses acid, liquid nitrogen, and even injected antibiotics to treat recalcitrant warts, homeopathy provides very effective and noninvasive, nonpainful treatments of them. The majority of hard, elevated, corny warts respond to *Antimonium Crudum*.

Potency and Dosage: For hard, elevated, corny warts, give Antimonium crudum in potencies of 6c to 15c (approximately 12x to 30x on the American decimal scale) in dosages of 5 1-grain tablets twice daily until symptoms subside.

For plantar warts (verrucas), quite common among athletes who share locker room facilities, Antimonium crudum is also exceptionally useful. Plantar warts are flat. But a side view would show a wart shaped much like an ice cream cone, with the pointed end penetrating deeply into the tissues of the foot. Here, the wart presses against sensitive nerves and creates pain. If the surface of the wart is yellowish and/or bleeds easily, and produces a characteristic pricking pain as if a needle were pressing into the foot, homeopathic *Nitric Acid* in internal potency should be given.

Potency and Dosage: Use 12x or 6c. One dose daily, taken together with Antimonium crudum as above, should relieve the condition within a short time.

One of the most difficult types of warts for standard medicine to treat are those appearing under and around the fingernails. Warts appearing under the nails are called *subungual* warts; those surrounding the nails but not beneath are called *periungual* qualified warts.

Causticum is almost a specific treatment for subungual warts.

Potency and Dosage: Give Causticum in either 12x or 6c potency in twice-daily doses of 5 1-grain tablets.

For periungual warts, the remedy of choice is *Graphites,* which appears to be nearly as specific to this type of wart as Causticum to subungual. The periungual wart is hard, horny, and fissured, giving its surface a rough, almost chapped appearance.

Potency and Dosage: Graphites in 3x, 6x or 3c potencies in twice-daily doses of 5 1-grain tablets. Alternate Antimonium crudum in either 12x–30x or 6c–15c potencies with Graphites once or twice daily. Graphites tincture may be applied directly onto the wart, 1 to 2 drops once or twice daily, in addition to taking graphites tablets internally.

CHAPTER ELEVEN

SOFT-TISSUE INJURIES

Topics Covered

Abrasions
Incisions, Lacerations, and Punctures

Abrasions

Any injury that scrapes away the uppermost layer of skin, exposing the underlying tissues to bacteria and possible infection, is called an abrasion. From the jogger who tumbles and scrapes hands or knees against the pavement, to the youthful baseball player who slides into base, abrasions are a common occurrence. Though they are often minor, the greatest danger that can come as a result of an abrasion is the threat of infection, by way of foreign matter that may enter the wound.

The immediate treatment for abrasion injuries is to thoroughly cleanse the injury of all surface dirt, and to remove any material that may have become embedded in the underlying tissues. This is best accomplished by washing the wound thoroughly with bland soap and water; work *from the center of the wound outward*, so as not to introduce additional foreign matter and bacteria from the surrounding healthy skin into the wound. Be observant and remove any embedded material. In especially severe abrasions where dirt, gravel, sand, or glass have become embedded, a qualified health care professional should be consulted.

HOMEOPATHIC TREATMENT
Calendula Succus
Nonalcoholic Calendula
Calendula Tincture

Following a careful cleansing, **Calendula Succus, Nonalcoholic Calendula,** or a 1:5 dilution of **Calendula Tincture** should be applied. Calendula succus contains only a small percentage of ethyl alcohol to preserve the fresh plant juice. Nonalcoholic Calendula is a mixture of the fresh plant juice in glycerin and purified water. Therefore, neither of these two excellent wound-healing products requires dilution. But, due to the high alcohol content of Calendula tincture, this product is best applied following its dilution of one part Calendula tincture to five parts of water.

Calendula is without question one of the most effective cleansing agents and healers of all types of wounds. Made from the juice of the African marigold plant, Calendula is not antiseptic but aseptic; it does not directly destroy bacteria, but bacteria cannot flourish in its presence. Calendula prevents infection by inhibiting bacterial growth, and it constricts blood vessels through a hemostatic or styptic quality that slows down bleeding and stops it in most cases where the bleeding is no more than superficial.

Incisions, Lacerations, and Punctures

Besides abrasions there are three other types of soft tissue injuries that figure less prominently in sports injuries: incisions, lacerations, and punctures.

Incised wounds are clean, relatively straight wounds which penetrate the skin's surface as would a knife. Incised wounds vary from those involving little tissue damage, and only minor to moderate bleeding, to the most severe, where the deepest substructures of the tissues are involved:

muscles, connective structures (tendons and ligaments), and nerves. Deeply incised wounds, such that white or yellowish fatty tissue shows, should always be evaluated and treated by a health care professional. Special treatment is also required if a wound is especially jagged and the edges do not "fit" well together.

Lacerations exceed incised wounds in the extent of their traumatic damage to underlying tissue structures. Lacerations are jagged and irregular, appearing quite literally as though the skin had been torn apart. Subsurface fatty tissue (yellow, white, or yellowish-white) may be exposed; larger blood vessels and even arteries may be damaged. Because of the extent of the tissue damage, lacerations provide a greater possibility for infection than do incised wounds, placing them perhaps on a par with puncture wounds in this respect.

Puncture wounds also occur in sporting competitions, although far less commonly today than in years past.

A puncture is any small wound produced when a sharply pointed object is driven into the skin. Because a puncture penetrates into the deepest tissues, the danger of infection is greatly enhanced. Penetrating objects may carry bacteria from the skin's surface or from the object itself.

Recent studies conducted at several major universities and medical institutions have demonstrated that traditionally used antiseptics meant to disinfect wounds actually retard healing. While they do disinfect the skin and tissues by attacking and destroying bacteria, these antiseptic products — iodine and its derivatives (Betadine, Providone, Acudyne, Mercurochrome, and Merthiolate to name a few) — damage and therefore retard the skin's natural ability to heal. Homeopathic aseptic medications do not damage the skin's cells and, therefore, promote rather than retard healing. Wounds treated with Calendula, Hypericum, or Hypercal will heal cleaner and up to two to three times faster, and with less possibility of secondary infection, than those treated with traditional antiseptics.

HOMEOPATHIC TREATMENT
Calendula
Hypericum
Hypercal
Ledum Palustre (Ledum Pal.)
Hepar Sulphuris Calcareum (Hepar Sulph.)
Pyrogen

Calendula, the first treatment to remember, has already been presented in its three forms. *Hypericum,* the homeopathic preparation of the herb St. John's wort, is the remedy of choice in lacerations. Due to the extent of substructure damage and therefore damage to nerves, Hypericum is the most appropriate remedy. Of course, should Hypericum be unavailable, Calendula should be readily substituted.

Hypericum is available only in an alcoholic tincture form, or combined as a hybrid with Calendula and called *Hypercal.* Because of its high ethyl alcohol content neither Hypericum tincture nor Hypercal should be applied to any open wound without dilution. A 1:5 dilution (1 part Hypericum tincture or Hypercal to 5 parts water) is appropriate in treating lacerations.

Puncture wounds require special consideration, and should never be treated lightly. The possibility of infection is ever-present, and the danger of tetanus high. Therefore, punctures should be encouraged to bleed, so that any bacteria and foreign material is encouraged to wash free of the wound.

Homeotherapeutics presents a treatment for puncture wounds that is indeed outstanding. *Ledum Pal.* (Ledum palustre), prepared from the herb marsh tea, is well known to homeopaths.

Surface treatment of puncture wounds has little benefit in stimulating healing or preventing infection. While the skin surrounding the site of injury may be treated with Calendula in its succus, tincture, or nonalcoholic forms – or Hypericum or Hypercal – the most appropriate treatment employs a 15-minute soak in Ledum pal., the tincture diluted 1:5 with water.

ADVISORY WARNING: In all puncture wounds the possibility of tetanus must be considered. Tetanus bacillus is anaerobic; it requires no oxygen to reproduce and cannot exist in the presence of oxygen. Every individual, and particularly all athletes, should be vaccinated against tetanus. In all cases of puncture injuries the medical record should be checked to see that a tetanus toxoid booster has been given within the past 5 years. A one day delay in a tetanus booster is acceptable, and allows the athlete time to check medical records and avoid the discomfort of unnecessary treatment.

Internal homeopathic prophylaxis against infection should always be considered in soft tissue injuries – in all open wounds and punctures as an adjunct to external treatment.

Calendula, Hypericum, and Ledum pal. have already been presented as effective external treatments in all open wounds. Taken by mouth in appropriate potencies, these same medicines work within the body, stimulating the body's own natural defenses against infection.

Calendula is a general prophylactic treatment in wounds which, by their extent and nature, demonstrate a possibility for infection. Hypericum in potency is especially beneficial in treating deeply incised wounds or lacerations, where nerve endings are either damaged or severed. Ledum pal. is most appropriately employed whenever the wounded part feels cold.

Potency and Dosage: In all the homeopathics noted above, potencies of 6x–30x or 3c–30c are appropriate. Dosage will vary depending upon the nature and extent of the injury and the degree of discomfort that may be involved. Generally, Calendula, Hypericum, or Ledum pal. are repeated every 2 hours in their lower potencies, or as pain occurs, and in their midrange potencies every 3 or 4 hours for a maximum of 9 doses.

Hepar Sulph. is a homeopathic mineral remedy. It is useful in any wound that forms or threatens to form pus, is a product of infection, or shows the traditional symptoms of inflammation: heat, redness, swelling, pain.

Potency and Dosage: To promote suppuration, Hepar sulph. is employed in its lower potencies (12x or below on the decimal scale; 6c and below on the centesimal scale). To eliminate infection the midrange potencies of 30x, 12c, or 15c should be employed. Standard dosage is 5 1-grain tablets to be given every 3 to 4 hours, as required.

Pyrogen is a homeopathic artificial septic pus derived from animal sources and introduced into homeopathic practice by British M.D.s. Pyrogen possesses excellent anti-infective properties and may well be considered in treating any wound that becomes infected. Used as a preventive agent and given internally, Pyrogen will frequently prevent infection.

Potency and Dosage: Pyrogen (also called Pyrogenium) may be used in potencies ranging from 12x–30x or 6c–30c or with benefit.

CHAPTER TWELVE

GENITOURINARY CONCERNS

Topics Covered

Testicular Torsion
Testicular Cancer
Penile Injuries
Epididymitis
Orchitis

Testicular Torsion

Testicular torsion is a rare but profound medical emergency, and is presented here to educate the sporting public.

This condition, while relatively rare, does occur in male athletes, most often in adolescent boys.

The testicles (or testes) develop in the abdominal cavity and shortly before birth pass downward through the inguinal canal to rest in the loose sack of skin called the scrotum. The testicles are oval-shaped structures encased in a tough, fibrous capsule that contains the fine tubes in which the sperm are formed. Nature in her infinite wisdom has made one testicle, usually the left, to hang lower than its neighbor, so that the two organs slide laterally whenever the man walks, runs, or sits, thereby avoiding a painful collision. On the outer, upper side of each testicle is a tightly coiled tube, the *epididymis,* that stores maturing sperm for a period of ten days. The epididymis is sometimes subject to inflammation—a topic which will be covered later in this chapter. From the epididymis runs the *vas deferens,* the main spermatic channel that runs up into the abdomen.

In testicular torsion, the testis twists on its chord, either spontaneously (without apparent cause) or through strenuous physical activity. This is one of the reasons that all male athletes should wear an athletic supporter. However, it is not at all uncommon for young and adolescent athletes to forego the jock strap in gym class and organized sporting activities, and almost certainly in playground activities. It is these situations where trouble may occur. The athletic supporter is designed to support the reproductive structures in the scrotum. During times of high temperature and the increase of body temperature resulting from athletic activities, the testicles move lower away from the body and are subsequently more prone to injury.

The immediate symptoms of testicular torsion are severe local pain without apparent cause (as a blow to the groin), nausea, and vomiting. Secondary symptoms will appear later—swelling of the scrotum and fever.

At the *first sign* of immediate symptoms, and before secondary symptoms appear, the victim should be taken to a physician or hospital emergency room. Most medical authorities recommend immediate surgical repair as the only course of treatment. If the correction does not occur within a few hours, the damage to the testicle is irreparable, and the testicle must be removed.

Testicular Cancer

Every young male between the ages of 15 and 35 should be aware of the possibility of testicular cancer. He should be as knowledgeable in self-examination of his testicles as are women today about the self-examination of their breasts.

Up until a decade ago, testicular cancer was one of the most common causes of death in males aged 29 to 35, and was 90% fatal. Now, with improved treatment methods and early detection, its cure rate is significantly greater.

John Donahue, M.D., Chairman of the Department of Urology at the Indiana University School of Medicine, recommends that all males, from early adolescence through early middle age, be thoroughly examined once a year for the earliest signs of trouble. He notes further that testicular tumors are rare among American blacks, black Africans, and Oriental males, but have a high frequency in white males. Dr. Donahue states additionally that all males with a history of sperm-duct inflammation (epididymitis) and testicular inflammation (orchitis), especially when due to mumps, are apparently the most prone to malignant tumors. The symptoms to watch for are:

1. There is a hard, painless mass or swelling within the testicle.
2. There is a feeling of pressure, or "dragging down" discomfort in the lower abdomen or testicle.

Fewer than 20% of all malignant tumors will produce pain.

Self-examination is simple and painless. It is best done while showering or bathing, when the testicles are hanging loosely away from the body. Each testicle should be carefully examined. Roll the testicle gently between the thumb and first two fingers. A normal testicle is oval (egg shaped) and has a firm, yet spongy (springy) consistency. Begin the examination high in the scrotum and trace the spermatic chord (vas deferens) downward to the testicle. Feel each structure and each testicle separately. Both testicles should be near identical images of one another as should the connecting structures. The testicle should be smooth-surfaced and spongy. If a lump or any unusual hardness is felt during the self-examination, the man should seek professional medical attention.

Parents of boys should instruct their sons in this self-examination procedure, as should all physical education instructors and athletic coaches in the schools. Parents must also understand and pass onto their sons the same understanding that there is nothing "evil" or "wrong" or "unclean" about this self-examination. Early detection is the key to survival, and any "I'm going to wait and see" attitude might be fatal.

I would urge all parents of adolescents, coaches, and physical education instructors to obtain information about testicular self-examination. In the UK, this can be obtained from:

BACUP
121/123 Charterhouse Street
London EC1M 6AA
Tel. (in London) 608 1661 or
(outside London) 0800 181199.

Penile Injuries

The penis surrounds the urethra, the long tube that extends from the urinary bladder to the outlet at the tip of the penis. The head of the penis, or *glans,* at birth is covered by a protective outer skin cover called the *foreskin.* Unlike men in the majority of Western, Middle Eastern, and Asian

Injuries to the penis are not uncommon in athletic activities, especially when athletic supporters are not worn. Questions as to the extent of any injury to the penis should receive a thorough medical evaluation. The most common injuries are zipper and bruising accidents.

HOMEOPATHIC TREATMENT
Calendula
Hypericum
Arnica Montana
Bellis Perennis

Zipper injuries are most common among very young sportsmen who, in their hurry to urinate and get back into the game, fail to tuck themselves away before zipping their fly.

Once the penis is removed from the zipper's teeth (a feat made easier by oiling or greasing the zipper), the wound should be cleaned with plain warm tap water, and either **Calendula** or **Hypericum** applied externally. A Band-Aid should then be applied. As the penis is especially sensitive because of its nerve-rich structure, Hypericum in homeopathic potency can be given orally. This treatment will quickly remove all pain.

Potency and Dosage: 6x–30x or 30c, 1 dose every 30 minutes for 3 doses, then 1 dose every 3 to 4 hours as needed until pain is gone.

The penis, unprotected by a supporter, is subject to bruising injuries. A bruise, or *contusion,* occurs when soft tissues and their capillaries are damaged, allowing blood and other fluids to leak into the surrounding tissue.

Arnica is a truly remarkable pain-relieving homeopathic remedy. Its ability to relieve pain is not due to any analgesic action of its own, but to its ability to rapidly heal damaged tissue and blood vessels. Arnica's rather amazing powers have been well known by European rock and mountain climbers for years and they are seldom without a supply in homeopathic potency.

Potency and Dosage: 6x–30c or 30c, 1 dose every 30 minutes for 3 doses, then 1 dose every 3 to 4 hours as needed for pain.

Bellis Perennis is the homeopathic name for a trituration of the common daisy. One would scarcely expect such a beautiful and delicate flower to produce a powerful bruise-relieving medicine.

Bellis perennis acts on the muscular tissues and the fibers of the blood vessels to produce a rapid, pleasant healing.

Potency and Dosage: Bellis is best used in low potencies (3x, 6x, and 3c), 1 dose every 1 to 2 hours as required until a noticeable reduction in outward symptoms occurs.

Epididymitis

Epididymitis is the medical term for a localized inflammation of the sperm duct. The location and purpose of the *epididymis* have already been discussed at the beginning of this chapter.

There are two types of epididymitis: *acute bacterial* and *nonbacterial.* Occasionally, bacterial epididymitis can also develop into a *chronic recurrent bacterial* form. In this condition, examination reveals swelling and marked tenderness of one portion or along the entire organ.

HOMEOPATHIC TREATMENT
Belladonna
Clematis
Hamamelis
Pulsatilla

Belladonna, in homeopathic potency, is prepared from the plant, the deadly nightshade. Its Keynote symptoms are:

1. There is great sensitivity to touch or pressure.
2. There is intolerance of pain.
3. Pain comes on suddenly and may disappear as suddenly.
4. (A "Key" symptom:) There is extreme *localization* of the site of pain.

Potency and Dosage: 6x–30x or 30c, 1 dose every 3 to 4 hours as required.

Clematis has the following Keynote symptoms:

1. The epididymis is greatly swollen.
2. Pain is especially acute from pressure.
3. The testicle feels drawn up and sensitive; pain may be felt along the spermatic chord, especially along the right.

Potency and Dosage: 6x–30x or 30c, 1 dose every 3 to 4 hours as required.

Hamamelis, the homeopathic preparation from the herb witch hazel, produces as its main Keynote symptom exquisite soreness, and a dull aching pain in the testicle, and along the spermatic chord.

Potency and Dosage: 6x–30x or 30c, 1 dose every 3 to 4 hours as required for relief.

Pulsatilla, from the wind flower, is one of the most highly regarded remedies in the homeopathic *Materia Medica* for epididymitis. Keynote symptoms follow:

1. The testicle feels drawn up and retracted.
2. The epididymis is enlarged, swollen and sensitive to pressure.
3. Dragging pains occur along the spermatic chord.
4. Pain from the site of inflammation shooting downward into the thigh is a special "Key" symptom.

Potency and Dosage: 6x–30x or 30c, 1 dose every 3 to 4 hours as required to relieve pain.

Orchitis

Orchitis is an inflammation of the testicle and usually the complication of a urinary tract infection or prostatitis (inflammation of the prostate gland) or urethritis (inflammation of the urethra). It may at times appear following the sexually transmitted disease gonorrhea. An inflammation occurring simultaneously in both the testicle and epididymis is called *Epididymo-orchitis*.

HOMEOPATHIC TREATMENT
Clematis
Gelsemium
Hamamelis
Pulsatilla
Rhododendron
Spongia

The remedies **Clematis, Hamamelis,** and **Pulsatilla** have already been presented. Treatment with these homeopathic remedies is the same in orchitis as in epididymitis, Keynote symptoms agreeing. Potency and dosage of the remedies are the same.

Gelsemium, a remedy prepared from the yellow jasmine flower, has received high praise from many homeopathic practitioners as a superior remedy in orchitis of gonorrheal origin. In Gelsemium the orchitis may also come on from a sudden exposure to cold dampness.

Potency and Dosage: Preferred potency is 30x or 30c, 1 dose every 3 to 4 hours as required. The remedy should be stopped after a maximum of 9 doses, or as soon as there is a noticeable reversal in the condition.

Rhododendron appears to be an excellent remedy in orchitis of a chronic nature, where the testis is swollen and painful, and the "Key" Keynote symptom, the testicle feels as if it is being crushed, is present.

Potency and Dosage: Preferred potency is 30x or 30c, 1 dose every 3 to

4 hours as required. The remedy should be stopped after a maximum of 9 doses, or as soon as there is a noticeable reversal in the condition.

Spongia is a remedy unfortunately not often found in lay practitioner's kit. Spongia has an especially good reputation in orchitis, especially the chronic form, and as well in epididymitis where the following Keynote symptoms are present:

1. There are hardness and swelling of the testicle.
2. There is squeezing pain.
3. The spermatic chord is swollen and painful; pains dart along the chord.

Potency and Dosage: The midrange (30x or 30c) potencies are preferred, 1 dose every 3 to 4 hours, for a maximum of 9 doses. In certain cases of orchitis, Spongia will follow Hamamelis or Pulsatilla well and may be required to totally resolve the case.

APPENDIX

USEFUL INFORMATION

Homeopathic Organizations

United Kingdom

Homeopathy is available on the NHS if your doctor has also qualified as a homeopath; alternatively he can refer you. For a list of homeopathic doctors send an SAE to:

The British Homeopathic
  Association
27a Devonshire Street
London NW1 1RJ
(01-935 2163)

For a register of non-medically qualified homoeopaths (i.e., without orthodox medical qualifications) send an SAE to:

The Society of Homeopaths
2 Artizan Road
Northampton NN1 4HU
(0604 21400)

Australia
Australian Homeopathic
  Association
c/o 16a Edward Street
Gordon
New South Wales 2027

New Zealand
New Zealand Homeopathic
  Society
PO Box 2939
Auckland

Suppliers of Homeopathic Remedies in the UK

Ainsworth's
38 New Cavendish Street
London
W1M 7LH
Tel. 01 935 5330

Freeman's
7 Eaglesham Road
Clarkston
Glasgow
Tel. 041 644 1165

The Galens Pharmacy
1 South Terrace
South Street
Dorchester
Dorset
Tel. 0305 63996

E. Gould & Son Ltd
14 Crowndale Road
London
NW1 1TT
Tel. 01 388 4752

Helios Homoeopathic Pharmacies
92 Camden Road
Tunbridge Wells
Kent
TN1 2QP
Tel. 0892 36393

A. Nelson & Co. Ltd
5 Endeavour Way
London
SW19
Tel. 01 946 8527

Introductory Reading

Homoeopathy: Medicine of the New Man George Vithoulkas, Thorsons.

Everybody's Guide to Homoeopathic Medicine Stephen Cummings and Dana Ullman, Gollancz.

Homoeopathy: Medicine for the 21st Century Dana Ullman, Thorsons.

Professional Reading

The Science of Homoeopathy George Vithoulkas, Thorsons.

Studies in Materia Medica D M Gibson, Beaconsfield.

The Organon of the Rational Art of Healing Samuel Hahnemann, Gollancz.

Homoeopathic Drug Pictures Margaret Tyler, Health Science Press.

Principal Sources of Information For This Book

Charles E. Wheeler, M.D., *An Introduction to the Principles and Practice of Homeopathy,* 3d ed. (N. Devon: Health Science Press, 1948).

William Boericke, M.D., *Materia Medica with Repertory,* Calcutta, Sett Dey & Company, 1976).

E. B. Nash, M.D., *Leaders in Homeopathic Therapeutics,* (Calcutta, Sett Dey & Company, 1959).

W. A. Dewey, M.D., *Practical Homeopathic Therapeutics,* 3d ed. (New Delhi: Jain Publishing Company, 1981).

M. L. Tyler, M.D. (Brux.), *Homeopathic Drug Pictures,* 3d ed. (Devon: Bradford, Holsworthy, 1952).

Dr. Med. P. Hamalcik, ed., *Biologische Medizin,* (Baden-Baden, West Germany: Aurelia-Verlag GmbH).

INDEX